Clinical Applications of Music Therapy in Developmental Disability, Paediatrics and Neurology

of related interest

Clinical Applications of Music Therapy in Psychiatry
Edited by Tony Wigram and Jos De Backer
ISBN 1 85302 733 2

Music Therapy in Health and Education
Edited by Margaret Heal and Tony Wigram
ISBN 1 85302 175 X

Music Therapy in Context
Music, Meaning and Relationship
Mercedes Pavlicevic
ISBN 1 85302 434 1

Music Therapy Research and Practice in Medicine
From Out of the Silence
David Aldridge
ISBN 1 85302 296 9

Clinical Applications of Music Therapy in Developmental Disability, Paediatrics and Neurology

Edited by Tony Wigram and Jos De Backer

Foreword by Colwyn Trevarthen

Jessica Kingsley Publishers
London and Philadelphia

The extract on pp.130–1 from *Snow Falling on Cedars,* by David Guterson is reproduced by kind permission of Bloomsbury Publishers, UK, and Harcourt Brace Inc.

First published in the United Kingdom in 1999 by
Jessica Kingsley Publishers Ltd,
116 Pentonville Road,
London N1 9JB, England
and
325 Chestnut Street
Philadelphia, PA 19106, USA.

www.jkp.com

Copyright © 1999 Jessica Kingsley Publishers.

Library of Congress Cataloging in Publication Data
A CIP catalog record for this book is available from the Library of Congress

British Library Cataloguing in Publication Data
Clinical applications of music therapy in developmental disability, paediatrics and neurology
1.Music therapy
I.Wigram, Tony II.De Backer, Jos
615.8'5154

ISBN 1-85302-734-0

Printed and Bound in Great Britain by
Athenaeum Press, Gateshead, Tyne and Wear

Contents

How Music Heals

Colwyn Trevarthen

The musicality of moving is an innate capacity of our brain and body, of a mind built to generate, imagine, feel emotional about, remember and recognize impulses and narratives of movement. With this complex vitality, human consciousness is also given a greatly enriched power of sympathy for the impulses that escape out of other humans' minds, signalled in their movements. As music gives expression to intrinsic pulses in the brain – the beats, rhythms, phrases and cyclic narratives – these time patterns carry affecting messages. They transmit intimate information about the inner emotional life of our interacting minds.

We have much new evidence on the biological origins of our musicality, from research on the preferential attentions even newborns pay to the melodies and time patterns of a mother's speech and song, and from the precision and affecting quality of infants' participation in vocal and gestural performances with playmates. This communication is not just for fun. Infants are responsive to the musicality of maternal expression as part of their adaptations to co-operate with and benefit from the strong messages of care, concern and love that a mother intuitively presents. Soon the infant is sharing curiosity, becoming observant of the ways things in the world are used by interested and friendly company. The Papoušeks, who have done much to reveal the nature of innate human musical skills, describe the mother's specially attentive behaviour as 'intuitive parenting'. They conclude it is the essential external regulator of the child's cognitive development, as well as being the emotional regulator of inner states of arousal and physiological maintenance. Non-verbal patterns of protoconversations and games with infants, which prove the shared sense of time between adult and infant, clearly serve in cultural learning and, specifically, in the awareness and learning of natural, conversational language. Daniel Stern has pioneered a theory of the infant's dynamic emotions and has described how the mother helps develop these into narratives of the experiencing self, giving the infant confirmation of consciousness and the will to live, by reflecting, or, as he puts it, 'attuning to' the inner trans-modal or multi-sensory impulses of moving and noticing. He and his colleagues have microanalysed the delicate timing and synchronizing of mother–infant exchanges. This work supports both a theory of self-awareness emerging in an attachment relationship, and a formula for sensitive therapeutic practices that may give vital support, without verbal or cold-reasoned interpretation of the inner processes in minds.

When we are healthy we attend and learn together, and we become easily committed in elaborate co-operative enterprises. As children we were supported in our purposes and discoveries through the appreciation of our interest and activity by older, more experienced, companions. In sickness we can be lifted up and given courage and relief from pain and fear by sharing vitality with the feelings and ideas of compassionate friends. They give us new interest in what is happening around us. Just as the vitality of music is essential in joyful celebrations, so taking part in music has the power to make well. Music is therapeutic because it attunes to the essential efforts that the mind makes to regulate the body, both in its inner processes and in its purposeful engagements with the objects of the world, and with other people. It is a most direct way of engaging the human need to be sympathized with – to have what is going on inside appreciated by another who may give aid and encouragement.

This collection of papers celebrates the sense of achievement shared by an international group of music therapists. Some describe how they have worked with frail and suffering newborns or brain-damaged patients being kept alive by intensive medical care. Others have been able to communicate with seriously mentally and emotionally disturbed youngsters, or children with an incurable disease and facing an early death.

Music therapy for human beings who are very immature, damaged, very old or gravely handicapped brings direct support for the irreducible core of human life, the central source of rhythms that seeks to make the body do things, that generates awareness of a body-centred world in which there are places to go and things to be done. It stimulates the need every human being has for perceptive, if not always kindly, company – for partners in moving, noticing and understanding. The emotions or motivating qualities of a person's acting and of being aware are shared by expressions of their every body part. They are rich and free in musical forms: in the unaided singing of the voice, in the expressive movements of the lips and tongue playing a wind instrument, and in the gestures of the hands, which can be made to sing and speak with the aid of instruments that sound to the beat of a limb or to a finger's touch.

Music can heal, but recognition of this has not been easily won. For dedicated music therapists it has been a long struggle. But now music therapy is gaining an increasing respect of doctors responsible for care of the most difficult patients. The medical world is a powerfully regulated one. Its traditions focus on treatment of the needs of the physical, chemical, somatic human being. Great strides in treatment of diseases, brilliant pharmacological and surgical achievements, the coupling of clever machines with vital functions to give artificial support, or to achieve physical imaging of vital, and even mental events, all of modern medicine gives confidence in the science of the body. What a musician might contribute to diagnosis and treatment of the seriously ill with his or her ephemeral communications must seem trivial, and to suggest that music should play a central part in management of extremely serious, life-threatening conditions may appear sentimental and irresponsible. And yet, time and time again doctors treating the physical body have had to acknowledge that their work has been supported significantly by changes in a patient's emotional state, awareness of life and will to live that have been caused by the companionship of communicating with a musically able and clinically sensitive therapist.

That the vital processes of premature newborns can be regulated by the sounds of the human voice is no longer surprising in the light of convincing evidence that in the last trimester a foetus can learn to recognize the sounds of the mother's voice. Research on the sensitivity of very young infants to the rhythmic and melodic dimensions of maternal speech, and to its emotional tone, convincingly demonstrates that we are born ready to engage with 'communicative musicality' of conversation. Mary Catherine Bateson described 'protoconversation' with a two-month-old as both the foundation for language and for 'ritual healing practices'. Healing results from aid that fights a disease process or that restores life functions. The power of communication to change a state of withdrawal and agitation into one of active recovery in which the control of autonomic state, emotional calming, resistance to pain and readiness to communicate and co-operate with caregivers are improved may be easily seen when music therapy has its full effect.

This book offers case studies and analyses of experience and theory that give a convincing, empirically supported account of how participation in musical communication does help patients with grave, life-threatening illnesses, transforming serious physiological dysregulations and emotional frailty. Contributors have worked with premature infants in intensive care, children with terminal illness, autism, physical or mental handicap, an abused child, emotionally disturbed teenagers, adults with neurological illness. All demonstrate how improvements can be elicited by sympathetic encouragement of musical experience and participation in musical improvisation, either with instruments or by singing. Music can give a guide to more skilled action, engage the emotions and give them coherence, develop a patient's sense of self-determination, and make a verbal narrative through which suffering or isolation may be articulated and accurately perceived within an understanding companionship. There are expert explanations of how music therapy should be planned and monitored, how it can be used for discriminating assessment of complex disorders of emotionality and communication, and how the work of trainee music therapists should be supervised. There are many beautiful and instructive examples from carefully recorded case studies. Undoubtedly, this collection will help establish effective therapy in which client-centred, interactive and creative use of music is employed by skilled and clinically sophisticated musicians. It makes the healing power of music clear.

PART ONE

Paediatrics

CHAPTER I

A Song of Life

Improvised Songs with Children with Cancer and Serious Blood Disorders

Ann Turry

> I'm just lying here all alone
> Got no place to call my own
> I can't explain the way I feel
> But you know my pain is real
> This is the worst time in my life
> But I can't give up the fight
> I've gotta find my way right through
> This endless night...

This chapter focuses on the use of improvised songs as a means of helping children to cope with the experience of a life-threatening or chronic disease. Issues related to illness and hospitalization, the impact of illness on normal childhood development and the effect on family members and the extended community will be delineated. The application of clinical improvisation within different settings and circumstances will be described. Aspects of Creative Music Therapy which are particularly relevant for this population will be presented and the importance of creativity, spontaneity and relationship will be emphasized as a theme.

While one focus of this chapter endeavours to outline a theoretical approach for this work and is primarily academic, there is another equally important aim: to introduce to the reader the stories and songs of children who face serious illness. In order to fully appreciate the power of music therapy in this setting, it is important to describe what it is like to undergo extensive medical treatment and hospitalization and to cope with the implications of living with a serious or life-threatening disease. The children in this chapter are different ages, come from various backgrounds and cultures and have different diagnoses. And the situations in which music therapy sessions occur are different. But what is common throughout is that all of them use the medium of musical improvisation to convey their thoughts and feelings – they relate their stories through their songs and tell us in a deep way what it's like to hurt or to want to go home. Within these songs are the voices of children and we hear their pain, their fears, their anger, their love and their courage.

Psychosocial aspects of illness

A child diagnosed with a life-threatening or chronic illness is confronted with a multitude of stresses and challenges. The initial hospitalization admission can be dramatic, long and confusing to both the child and the family. Families spend the first few days acclimatizing to a new environment and adjusting to the impact of the diagnosis. Procedures, tests and surgery seem to occur in a sequence of blurred days and there is often a sense of anxiety as the family waits to hear the differential diagnosis that will determine the extent and severity of the disease. Dramatic side effects from the initial medications or unanticipated medical crises may add to the level of acute distress. The rooms can be crowded and families may have little space. Meetings with the team (physicians, nurses, social workers, creative arts therapists) may feel overwhelming and confusing to parents as the treatment plan is reviewed and unfamiliar nomenclature is introduced. Words like 'prognosis', 'radiation', 'morbidity', 'surgery' and 'chemotherapy' may be used in the context of a small child who was out playing ball last week before the headaches or bruises began to appear. Sleep patterns are interrupted frequently as nurses must come in and out of the room throughout the night to adjust medications or take vital signs. A multitude of visitors is common and many of these visitors can be emotional or anxious, adding to the overall feeling of fear, anger or confusion in the atmosphere. Parents must contend with what to tell family members, how to communicate with their child's school and how to handle the immediate surge of community reaction.

The child can be overwhelmed with confusing sensory input and emotional reactions. They may feel sick due to the beginning of treatment or they may be in a lot of pain. They are often attached to an intravenous drip and a pole which they must push around if they are able to ambulate, or they may not be able to leave their beds at all. The days seem filled with endless pokes, squeezes, pinches from needles and awful-tasting medicine. The child may be too young to understand what is happening or why it is happening – it may seem like a punishment or an assault. The pervasive feelings of distress are absorbed, though intellectual understanding may not accompany the feeling, resulting in increased fear and confusion. In response to this extreme situation, a child may withdraw, regress or act out.

These experiences can define the early days of living with a life-threatening or chronic illness. Overwhelming and traumatic moments which seem unbearably long at times pass in a blur as a family's life is changed forever.

Issues of hospitalization

In recent years The Association for the Care of Children in Hospitals and the Child Life Council in the United States has significantly raised awareness of the impact of hospitalization on normal childhood development. Potential issues related to hospitalization and illness and appropriate coping strategies and interventions have been well documented in the current literature by paediatricians, psychologists, nurses and child life specialists (Bearison and Mulhern 1994; Sanger, Copeland and Davidson 1991; Spirito, Stark and Tye 1994). Issues and circumstances, both general and specific to cancer, that may influence a child's adaptive adjustment to their illness include:

- extended stays in the hospital
- separations from friends and family members
- restriction of movement or physical activity
- loss of control and feelings of powerlessness
- painful and intrusive medical procedures
- noxious side effects from medical treatment (i.e., nausea, pain, fatigue, etc.)
- misunderstanding of nature of illness and cause of disease
- confrontation with multiple losses on different levels
- potential exacerbation of pre-morbid conflicts or psychopathology
- potential changes in appearance or disfigurement
- fear of death/annihilation.

Some of the issues are overt and dramatic (i.e., the immediate perceived threat of death upon diagnosis, painful procedures associated with treatment or the loss of hair due to chemotherapy), while others are more subtle yet can be debilitating or demoralizing (i.e., increased dependence upon others or loss of control). The potential for the manifestation of specific issues depends upon a number of factors which include: the specific illness, prognosis and treatment protocol; a child's developmental level and temperament; the availability and quality of support; a child's coping style and strategies; and their threshold for pain and distress.

Similar to children with cancer, children who suffer from a chronic blood disorder can be hospitalized and undergo invasive medical procedures frequently. But there are distinct differences in the progression of these diseases and their psychosocial impact. Children with sickle-cell anaemia or other types of blood disorders may lead apparently 'normal' lives, yet the disease impacts their routine and activities in powerful and insidious ways. Studies examining the emotional adjustment of children with sickle cell reveal the potential for emotional immaturity, behavioural problems, low self-esteem and disturbances in body image and sexuality (Brown *et al.* 1995).

Developmental concerns

A child's normal pace of development may be challenged or interrupted by the rigours of illness and treatment. Regression is common in children who are confronted with acute distress. Toddlers who have recently mastered potty training may lose the ability to control their bladder or bowels and need nappies, others may lose the ability to separate from their caretakers and older patients who have mastered more sophisticated forms of coping or conceptualization may regress back to more immature levels of functioning (i.e., crying, tantrums, concrete thinking, etc.). It is imperative to acknowledge the impact of illness on normal childhood development and to emphasize the need for developmentally-based interventions. The objective is to help children to maintain as normal a developmental progression as possible despite the limitations and challenges of the illness.

The effect on family members

The impact of a diagnosis of cancer extends beyond the patient and affects the family and community on a variety of levels (Kazak *et al.* 1995; Sales

1991; Walco, Lewis and Schmerl 1994). In addition to their experience in relation to the patient, family members undergo their own unique processes in coming to terms with the illness. Cancer happens to the whole family – to the patient whose life and routine is irrevocably changed from the moment of diagnosis; to the parents who may be devastated but need to mobilize their resources in order to maintain their role of caretakers of the family; to the siblings who may be confused, angry or sad; and to the extended family members and significant others in the community who try to provide support while dealing with their own responses and emotions. All of these relationships influence each other in an ongoing cycle of reaction and adjustment. '…an individual with a chronic illness affects many individuals in the family, and family reactions have a substantial impact on the adjustment of the individual' (Walco, Lewis and Schmerl 1994, p.269).

One of the primary goals of psychosocial intervention is to help each family to cope as effectively as is possible given their abilities, resources and specific circumstances. It is important to approach each family with an attitude of receptivity and respect for their individual family system, coping and defence styles, and interactive patterns.

Music therapy

In recent years there has been increasing interest in, and awareness of, the efficacy of music therapy with hospitalized children. Fagen (1982) wrote about its effect on anxiety and fear in terminally ill children and Brodsky (1989) described its use with children in isolation for bone marrow transplant. McDonnell (1983) wrote about its effectiveness in meeting the emotional needs of hospitalized children and Standley and Hanser (1995) provided an overview of music therapy applications and research in paediatric oncology. In 1997 Loewy gathered clinicians together to engage in a focused dialogue about music therapy and paediatric pain management at the First National Music Therapy and Pediatric Pain Symposium, held in New York City. As a result of this symposium the first book on paediatric pain management and music therapy was published (Loewy 1997).

Techniques that have been identified in the literature include: music listening, songwriting, lyric substitution/analysis and improvisation. As a Nordoff–Robbins-trained music therapist, I am deeply influenced by the tenets of Creative Music Therapy. The principles underlying this approach are extremely relevant for children facing a life-threatening or chronic illness and I have found that clinical improvisation is a powerful and effective approach to address the many needs of this emotionally challenging population.

Clinical improvisation

Due to its inherently dynamic nature, clinical improvisation is an ideal medium for a setting in which profound changes can occur from moment to moment. Given the range of situations in which music therapy sessions take place in the medical setting, it is important to tailor the nature of the musical intervention to fit the needs of moment – whether a therapist is working at the side of the bed of a thirteen-year-old who is dying, intervening in the treatment room with a screaming seven-year-old, or meeting a frightened three-year-old who is in the hospital for the first time. Through clinical improvisation, a therapist can respond to the individuality of the child, taking cues from them – whether musical, verbal, behavioural or emotional – to create the foundation of the music and the relationship. Through responsiveness to the child and the intentional and sensitive use of musical elements, a therapist can connect to a child's experience and establish rapport.

Nordoff and Robbins (1977) wrote about creating a musical and emotional environment. Within the freedom of clinical improvisation, a therapist is able to 'respond musically to what [a child's] presence communicates: his bearing; facial expression; his glance;…his movements; his mood… [The] aim is to communicate with him as he is' (p.93). Each situation requires flexibility and creativity in order to establish meaningful and supportive contact with the child.

Active music making and improvisation provide the foundation for therapeutic contact from which relationships can be developed and specific needs addressed. The mutual co-activity of improvisation inspires a sense of shared experience – of joyous, spontaneous and playful interaction. Pavlicevic (1997) reminds us that music appeals to the whole person – to those aspects which may be 'sick' and yet also to those human capacities in us for creativity and growth. The essence of the musical experience – creativity, spontaneity, aesthetics – transcends the barriers of illness and physical limitation. A child's natural impulses toward development and engagement with others can be restored. Through the musical relationship, and, potentially, through activating the will of the child, a child's resources – strength, resilience, fortitude – can be mobilized to help withstand the rigours of the hospital. These principles of the Creative Music Therapy approach – relationship, responsiveness, spontaneity, mutuality and will – are particularly relevant for a medical setting that is unpredictable and can impart a sense of urgency to each moment. Sometimes, the goal of music therapy is to help a child manoeuvre or negotiate an intrusive experience such as an injection. In these instances it has been important to improvise music *for* the child rather than *with* the child. A therapist may support a child through music aimed to relax, soothe, empower or stimulate during these challenging situations. Musical choices are based on the relationship, observations of the child, the physical setting of the session and the immediate needs of the moment.

FORM

Barbara Sourkes (1995) writes: 'psychotherapy with the seriously ill child demands that unstructured associative communication be combined with highly focused interventions' (p.2). This approach is similar to that of the music therapist who reflects and structures a child's musical offerings and develops it into an aesthetic form. Form provides a sense of organization and stability. It is a safe and predictable means of interaction – a meeting ground for work. It 'provides the child with a structure he can understand and relate to – a sensory and emotional stimulation he can anticipate, and a recurring "space" in which he can respond' (Nordoff and Robbins 1977, p.102). Form – whether in the music or in the interaction in general – gives an experience a direction and a purpose. Once a sense of form and structure are established, a level of communication is created and the potential for intercommunication becomes possible. In working with seriously ill children, form and structure can be important pathways toward communication.

IMPROVISED SONGS

Improvised songs offer important forms for a child to explore feelings related to illness and hospitalization. The added element of lyrics introduces another level of expression that is clear and tangible. Songs offer avenues for processing a child's experience directly or metaphorically and can be an effective medium for addressing painful issues. Music intensifies the affect underlying the content of the lyrics and provides a safe structure into which impulses and feelings can be projected and contained. As the tension underlying emotional energy is released and dissipated, uncomfortable emotions – such as sadness, fear or anger – can be safely acknowledged and explored:

...song improvisations bring the child to a deeper level of awareness of his/her feelings and tolerance for their expression. Through the improvisation, the therapist can give permission and support to the child to express feelings that the child perceives as forbidden, dangerous, or overwhelming. The musical structure and the context of the song make it safer for the child to experience feelings kept out of consciousness because of their threatening nature. (Bruscia 1987, pp.378–379)

Music therapy in practice

Music therapy can be used in a variety of ways to help children to deal with the myriad challenges of illness. Sessions are conducted in the hospital and the outpatient clinic on an individual and group basis. Through active music making, a child is often intrinsically motivated toward interaction, play and engagement with their environment. In the treatment room music may be used to support and empower a child during an intravenous (IV) insertion or lumbar puncture. The dynamic nature of improvisation is ideal for use in the procedure room where the needs of the moment change suddenly and frequently. Music has been used with children who are dying to foster a sense of shared meaningful experience for the families and to offer opportunities to say goodbye. And siblings have written songs about their unique experiences as a brother or sister of a seriously ill child while bereaved siblings have used songwriting effectively to convey their sense of loss and recount their experience of the death. Music can be used throughout the treatment process to meet the changing needs of the child.

IN THE HOSPITAL

'Barbara's Song' (Figure 1.1) describes the feelings of a seven-year-old who is being treated for acute lymphocytic leukaemia. In her treatment she undergoes painful medical procedures, including spinal taps, IV insertions and injections. She is hospitalized every three weeks for chemotherapy infusion and comes to the clinic weekly for blood tests. When she gets a fever she must be hospitalized and kept in isolation until the fever or infection is resolved. Her school and daily routines are interrupted on a regular basis and if a friend has a cold, she cannot play with them. Her mother and father take turns staying with her in the hospital at night and her grandmother stays with her during the day so her parents can continue to work. During hospitalizations she does not see her elder brother and is away from her toys

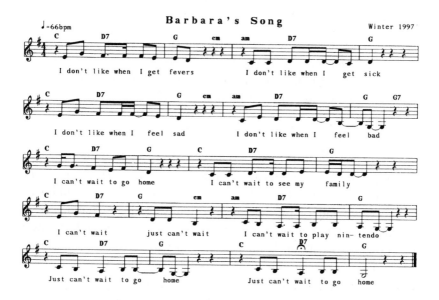

Figure 1.1 Barbara's Song

and games, such as Nintendo. She has lost her hair due to chemotherapy and often feels tired or nauseous due to medication. In her words, there is a lot not to like about her treatment.

The music of the song was developed mutually. As Barbara spoke about the aspects of her illness she did not like, I improvised a musical structure around the words, taking into consideration the melodic contour of her inflection, the dynamic range of her voice and her physical presentation. As she spoke, she sat with her legs tucked under her on the hospital bed, taking up a small amount of space. She chose a small instrument to accompany the song (a little maraca) and spoke softly and tentatively.

The dynamic of the guitar was soft and the strum was gentle. I chose to use my fingers, rather than a pick, to strum the guitar and created a soft and continuous texture in order to match Barbara's small voice – which sounded even younger than her seven years. The form consists of a repeated melodic phrase and a diatonic harmonic progression. This simple form repeats throughout both the first and second verse.

It is often important for children to sing their songs on their own in order to express the identified feelings and take ownership of the stated feeling. 'Singing is a direct expression of the ego living simultaneously in its emotional life, its mental life, and in its physical vocal apparatus' (Nordoff and Robbins 1965, p.137). After Barbara sang the song once on her own, I joined her, in order to provide a sense of support and acceptance. At times, it is important for the therapist to sing with the child – especially after the child has sung alone – in order to reinforce the ego and provide grounding in the here-and-now through the relationship.

IN THE PROCEDURE ROOM

The alleviation of distress is a primary goal in the procedure room and improvisation has been effective in a number of ways. The therapist may make music with a child prior to a procedure, accompany the child during the procedure and/or provide an opportunity for improvisation after its completion. Improvisation can be used to prepare, engage and empower a child prior to a needle stick. Improvised songs may include 'I Am Brave' to bolster a sense of self-efficacy and confidence. A song such as 'I Hate Needles' can structure and direct a child's feelings into a creative and dynamic form as the energy underlying the cathexis dissipates and a sense of control and mastery is established. And improvisations can help a child to process, express and integrate their experience (Turry 1997). Each stage of the procedure poses different challenges and offers different possibilities for mastery and success.

Anthony was eight years old and in the hospital for a vaso-occlusive episode due to his sickle-cell disease. When I arrived with my guitar and instruments, Anthony was friendly and enthusiastic about music therapy. Immediately upon starting the session a nurse arrived and informed Anthony that he needed an IV drip inserted. Since Anthony's mother had left for work, I accompanied him to the procedure to provide emotional support. The procedure was long and painful. When children are repeatedly stuck with needles, their veins become weak and it is difficult to find access for blood or fluid exchange. During the procedure the medical staff reassured him that the stick was only a 'pinch', that it wouldn't hurt too much and that it would help him to feel better. He repeatedly pleaded with them to try the needle in his hand instead of his arm. After approximately twelve needle sticks in both his hand and arm, the nurse was finally able to find an accessible vein. Anthony was shaken by the experience and distraught as we returned to his room to continue the session. Intuitively, I brought the medical play doll (whose name is 'Sal'). It is common practice in hospital settings to provide children with medical 'dolls' and facilitate an opportunity for the child to replicate the procedure on the doll as a means of acting out their experiences and working through their feelings. I asked Anthony if he would like to create a 'hospital song' and a 15-minute-long improvisation ensued in which he recounted his experience in the procedure room in great detail. Within the form of the improvisation, we sang both antiphonally and together, role playing the doctor, nurse and himself. I played a 12-bar blues progression in E major on the guitar and he beat a drum enthusiastically (Figure 1.2).

The blues progression provided a predictable and repetitive harmonic form. The strum was active and rhythmic as I muted the strings with my right hand to create a syncopated groove. The dynamic was moderately loud. My intent was not to soothe or calm Anthony but to try to match what I perceived as the intensity of his emotional experience at that moment. I wanted the music to convey a sense of strength and fortitude (the active and rhythmic strum) and also provide him with the support needed to recount his experience (the predictability of the form). This melody acted as a general theme of the improvisation and we often sang this part together. In between this refrain, we improvised lyrics which described different aspects of the procedure (Figure 1.3).

These sections developed through antiphonal singing and seemed more of a musical dialogue. There was no clear melodic development or consistent form and the rhythm was less accurate when words were spoken. Because of

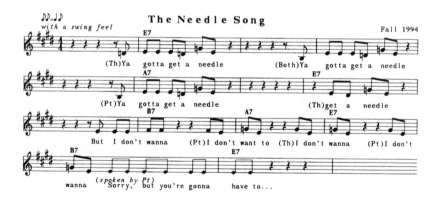

Figure 1.2 The Needle Song

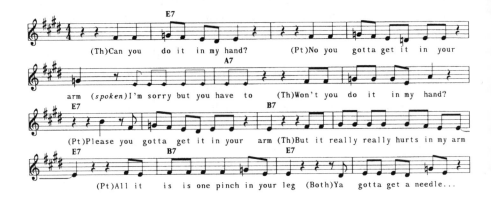

Figure 1.3

the clarity of the blues structure, we were able to expand the melodic line to accommodate our spontaneous musical impulses yet remain related to the overall form. The harmonic and rhythmic structure of the blues pattern provided the necessary foundation to freely explore musical intuitions yet return to the melodic theme as needed.

After this improvisation, during which the intensity of the feelings seemed to dissipate, we improvised a gentle song about how brave Sal, the medical doll, had been through this experience. At this point Anthony had begun to distance himself from the experience and project his feelings onto Sal. He began to minimize the intensity of the procedure and deny that the event had been painful or difficult. I felt it was important to support his efforts toward reasserting his defences. But it was equally important to validate that the procedure did, indeed, hurt and that he had survived and mastered the experience (Figure 1.4).

This second song was quiet and lyrical. The guitar strum was less active and the chords were sustained. The melody centred around E and the highest and longest note, G, was sung when affirming that the needle 'did' (or didn't)

Sal's Song

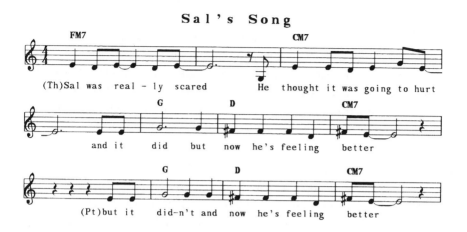

Figure 1.4 Sal's Song

hurt. The melody then descended downward to return and end on E. I played major seventh chords and the harmonic centre seemed ambiguous – the melody could be in the key of E minor yet the harmonic phrase ends on a CM7 chord (VIM7 in the key of E minor). There was no indication of a clear cadence which may have added to a sense of ambivalence around the statement. The lyrics were repetitive, rather than an ongoing dialogue, and aimed to affirm his success and mastery. We both sang more softly. An interesting observation to note is that when I made a conscious decision to sing very softly towards the end, Anthony ended the song. My decision to sing softly was a clinical one, made in order to evaluate how softly he could sing. I wanted to see how much he could contain and control his feeling and expression at this point. The fact that he ended the improvisation may have been an indication that this challenge was too much for him, that there was still a certain amount of tension related to his experience which needed to be released.

As a safe place is established in the music and the experience is recounted, a child's relationship to his environment is re-established. I refer to this process as reconstitution – a period in which ego is reinforced and the ability to cope is reasserted (Turry 1997). Anthony was able to use the improvisation to tell his story, reassert his defences and to reconstitute. Through expression, form and release he was able to move through his experience – he did not remain immobile in his helplessness. Within the mutually co-created structure of our improvisation, he was able to transform a threatening and overwhelming experience into one filled with spontaneity, meaning and purpose. He was living in the creative moment, meeting the moment and asserting his basic aliveness. He was having fun.

IN THE DYING PROCESS

A therapist may accompany a child through the dying process, using music as a means of connection and support during this life transition. The therapist sensitively observes and takes cues from the child and the family in the moment and in the context of the relationship to structure the contact and interventions. Often, family members are included in sessions during this time. These sessions can offer a means of expression for the human capacity towards growth and relationship, even in the face of physical deterioration. Music can support the patient's affirmations of life – a statement of 'I am here' – as they strike the cymbal quietly or tap the tambourine repeatedly while laying in bed, weak or semi-conscious. Each situation is unique and brings different challenges, yet within these challenges exists opportunity for shared experience and connection. 'Music therapy, with its emphases on personal contact and the value of the patient as a creative productive human being, has a significant role to play in the fostering of hope in the individual' (Aldridge 1996, p.232).

Aldridge writes about 'stimulating the awareness of living' (p.231) even when faced with death. This life energy may be the impetus for the child to reach out to touch the windchimes or turn towards the therapist as she sings quietly.

Dany was a five-year-old Egyptian boy who had Medulloblastoma, a brain tumour, and was in his last weeks of life. The treatment had failed, the tumour recurred and there was little else to do but keep him comfortable and treat the symptoms as they arose. His mother, father and two-year-old sister maintained a close vigil by his bed, moving into the hospital room in the final weeks. They were receptive to my presence and efforts with Dany. I had worked with Dany for fourteen months and a solid and trusting relationship existed between myself and all the family members. Dany spoke little English and the primary means of communication between myself and him had been musical.

As Dany's physical state declined, his ability to participate actively in music decreased, though he continued to make valiant efforts until he fell unconscious approximately one week before he died. I tailored the music to meet his changing needs, carefully re-evaluating my objectives each time I met with him to accommodate his deteriorating medical status. One day, after striking the cymbal as he lay in bed, Dany fell asleep holding the mallet firmly in his hand. His sleep was brief and as he awoke he reached for the cymbal and began to play. This gesture seemed a statement of his being and his need for continued interaction and acknowledgement – his need for continued life. Even in the face of death, Dany was able to maintain a growing, creative relationship. Prior to his final hospitalization, Dany was brought to the clinic and I met with him in an exam room. He sat on his mother's lap, slumped over and quiet. I felt a need to create something *for* Dany as it seemed unclear at the time what his potential for further interaction might be. It was an intuition on my part as I sat quietly with him and his mother, who appeared frightened and lost, rocked him gently and caressed his head. The song, though improvised, emerged in full form and it was never altered. I sang it to him each time I saw him and it became a ritual at the beginning or end of each session (Figure 1.5).

The intent behind the intuition was to improvise a song which reflected his gentle presence and could act as an acknowledgement of his impact on me. I was deeply moved by Dany and his continued efforts towards life and relationship. Shortly after he died, he lay in his mother's arms and I sang this song to him one last time. It was my way of saying goodbye to him and thanking him for all of our time together. It was my way of acknowledging

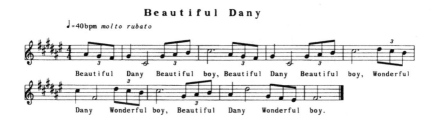

Figure 1.5 Beautiful Dany

my loss. It is difficult to know the actual effect that this song had on Dany. When the song was conceptualized he was already near the end of his life and he wasn't able to let me know. The song was improvised, in part, from an intuition based on clinical need in the moment. Yet the intuition was also based on personal feelings related to this situation and this particular moment. It is important to appreciate the conscious and unconscious motivations behind our interventions and intuitions in these delicate situations. Working with children who die is emotionally depleting and can arouse a myriad of responses. It is essential for those of us who work in this field to examine our feelings in relation to children and death and to observe how they influence the therapy process.

Children who come into the hospital with a serious illness are confronted with many challenges and stresses. Nothing can eradicate the intensity and potential trauma of this life event but music therapy can be effective in helping children to cope with these challenges. Through active music making and the therapist's conscious use of musical elements, initial rapport can be established and a child can feel heard and understood. Form provides a sense of structure and organization within a situation and can help a child to understand or process their experience. Clinical improvisation and songs offer avenues for the expression of thoughts and feelings while important issues are addressed sensitively and productively. Through expression, form and release, the underlying energy – or cathexis – can be regulated or dissipated and a sense of mastery and control can be restored.

Within an otherwise sterile and potentially threatening environment, sparks of life can be felt. In the creative moment a child's natural impulse toward playfulness, spontaneity and joy can be expressed and honoured.

> …And now that it has been a year
> I can see the end is near
> I kept giving it my best
> I think I passed the test
> The tunnel's end is in my sight
> And at last I see the light
> I finally found my way through
> This endless night.
>
> (David, age 20)

Glossary

Cathexis: invested energy in a mental representation – creates tension.

Clinical improvisation: a structure in which a therapist and a client or clients engage that is active, mutual, creative, spontaneous and free. Improvisation can be used throughout the assessment and treatment process.

Coping: the strategies an individual uses to deal with significant threat to his psychological stability. It does not carry with it the somewhat negative implications that can be associated with 'defence'.

> Coping can be thought of as consisting of two aspects, an externally directed one, judged for effectiveness in social terms, such as…the ability of the parent to participate in the care of his ill child and fulfill his other responsibilities, and an internally directed or defensive aspect, which serves to protect the individual from disruptive degrees of anxiety…
> (Chodoff, Friedman and Hamburg 1964, p.744)

Creative Music Therapy: an approach to music therapy developed by Paul Nordoff and Clive Robbins in which live, improvised music – generally played at the piano – is used to facilitate the therapeutic process. Initially, this approach was used with autistic and developmentally delayed children but in recent years it has been expanded to include clients of all types and with a variety of needs. CMT emphasizes musical aesthetics and the importance of mutuality and creativity.

Distress: the combination of pain and anxiety. A child's pain experience is intrinsically correlated to his level of anxiety. Neither element is mutually exclusive of the other and cannot be measured separately as they both continuously interact and influence the other.

Ego: the aspect of the personality which is able to separate fantasy from reality, internal from external, self from others. The centre of consciousness and rationality. It is in the ego that reality testing occurs.

Lumbar puncture/spinal tap: a procedure in which a needle is inserted between the bones of the spine and a sample of the cerebral spinal fluid is removed for analysis of the cells. This is a standard diagnostic procedure for children with leukaemia.

Medulloblastoma: a brain tumour located in the cerebellum. This is the second most common form of paediatric brain tumour and is usually treated with surgery, radiation and chemotherapy.

Reconstitution: a process in which the senses, emotions and ego functions are restored and reorganized after an intense emotional experience. During this process, re-engagement with others and the environment is achieved and the child's defences are either relaxed or reasserted. Previously aroused physiologic functions return to normal levels.

Sickle-cell anaemia: a hereditary haematological disorder which is characterized by chronic anaemia and episodes of vaso-occlusion produced by the 'sickling' of abnormally shaped red blood cells. Children are born with sickle cell and, at present, there is no cure.

Vaso-occlusive episode: an episode in which the red blood cells 'sickle' and occlude and prohibit oxygen from travelling to needed organs and areas of the body. These episodes occur in localized areas of the body and are characterized by extreme pain. Treatment generally requires hospitalization, pain medication and IV hydration.

Acknowledgements

I would like to thank David Marcus for his organizational skills and editorial suggestions for this chapter. I also want to thank and acknowledge my husband, Alan Turry, for his generous and consistent support and his guidance in delving deeper into the concepts of Nordoff–Robbins music therapy. Finally, I would like to acknowledge the children with whom I work – whose spirit and tenacity give life to this chapter and to my days at the hospital.

References

Aldridge, D. (1996) *Music Therapy Research and Practice in Medicine.* London: Jessica Kingsley Publishers.

Bearison, D.J. and Mulhern, R.K. (1994) *Pediatric Psychooncology: Psychological Perspectives on Children with Cancer.* New York and Oxford: Oxford University Press.

Brodsky, W. (1989) 'Music therapy as an intervention for children with cancer in isolation rooms.' *Music Therapy 8,* 1, 17–34.

Brown, R.T., Eckman, J., Baldwin, K., Buchanan, I. and Dingle, A.D. (1995) 'Protective aspects of adaptive behavior in children with sickle cell syndromes.' *Children's Health Care 24,* 4, 205–222.

Bruscia, K. (1987) *Improvisational Models of Music Therapy.* Springfield: Charles C. Thomas Publishers.

Chodoff, P., Friedman, S.B. and Hamburg, D.A. (1964) 'Stress, defenses and coping behavior: Observations in parents of children with malignant disease.' *American Journal of Psychiatry 120,* 743–749.

Fagen, T.S. (1982) 'Music therapy in the treatment of anxiety and fear in terminal pediatric patients.' *Music Therapy 2,* 1, 13–23.

Kazak, A.E., Boyer, B.A., Brophy, P., Johnson, K. and Scher, C.D. (1995) 'Parental perceptions of procedure-related distress and family adaptation in childhood Leukemia.' *Children's Health Care 24,* 3, 43–158.

Loewy, J.V. (ed) (1997) *Music Therapy and Pediatric Pain.* Cherry Hill: Jeffrey Books.

McDonnell, L. (1983) 'Music therapy: Meeting the psychosocial needs of hospitalized children.' *Children's Health Care 12,* 1, 29–33.

Nordoff, P. and Robbins, C. (1965) *Therapy in Music for Handicapped Children.* London: Victor Gollancz Ltd.

Nordoff, P. and Robbins, C. (1977) *Creative Music Therapy.* New York: The John Day Company.

Pavlicevic, M. (1997) *Music Therapy in Context.* London: Jessica Kingsley Publishers.

Sales, E. (1991) 'Psychosocial impact of the phase of cancer on the family: An updated review.' *Journal of Psychosocial Oncology 9,* 4, 1–18.

Sanger, M.S., Copeland, D.R. and Davidson, E.R. (1991) 'Psychosocial adjustment among pediatric cancer patients: A multidimensional assessment.' *Journal of Pediatric Psychology, 16,* 4, 463–474.

Sourkes, B. (1995) *Armfuls of Time: The Psychological Experience of the Child with a Life-Threatening Illness.* Pittsburgh: University of Pittsburgh Press.

Spirito, A., Stark, L.J. and Tye, V.L. (1994) 'Stressors and coping strategies described during hospitalization by chronically ill children.' *Journal of Clinical Child Psychology 23,* 3, 314–322.

Standley, J.M. and Hanser, S.B. (1995) 'Music therapy research and applications in pediatric oncology treatment.' *Journal of Pediatric Oncology Nursing 12,* 1, 3–8.

Turry, A.E. (1997) 'The use of clinical improvisation to alleviate procedural distress in young children.' In J.V. Loewy (ed.) *Music Therapy and Pediatric Pain.* Cherry Hill: Jeffrey Books.

Walco, G., Lewis, G. and Schmerl, L.T. (1994) 'Psychological aspects of coping with chronic illness.' In I.R. Shenker (ed.) *Adolescent Medicine.* Switzerland: Harwood Academic Publishers.

CHAPTER 2

Indications for the Inclusion of Music Therapy in the Care of Infants with Bronchopulmonary Dysplasia

Helen Shoemark

The Royal Children's Hospital, Melbourne, is the largest paediatric health centre in the southern hemisphere. The Neonatal Unit within it is a tertiary centre for premature and term infants with physical needs requiring complex medical or surgical intervention. Service delivery is based on the medical model, with primary care administered by nurses and all other services supplied on a referral basis only.

The clinical application of music therapy in the neonatal intensive care unit is still a new phenomenon. The programme at the Royal Childrens' Hospital, Melbourne, is the only one of its kind so far. This programme was commenced on the basis that music therapy has been successfully used elsewhere in the hospital with infants and children for more than eight years.

The research basis for this clinical programme includes the quantitative studies undertaken by American music therapists and nursing researchers concerned with the physiological impact of music and its efficacy in reducing stress on the infant (Burke *et al.* 1995; Caine 1992; Cassidy and Standley 1995; Kaminski and Hall 1996; Standley 1998; Standley and Moore 1995). It also draws on the infant psychiatry literature (Als 1986, 1992; Burns *et al.* 1994) for assessment and protocol. The underpinning philosophy is developmental because of the cultural context (Australian) and the context care in this setting – by developmental I mean concepts relating to the childhood development in the motor, cognitive, communication and social domains.

Much of the music therapy research seeks to demonstrate the safety and benefits of music for very low birth-weight premature infants. In American studies the central concern is to demonstrate how music can help to minimize the length of the hospital admission and promote early neurological development (Standley 1991). In Europe the concern is to promote the healthy relationship between mother and very low birth-weight infant (Nöcker-Ribaupierre 1996). At the Royal Children's Hospital, Melbourne, the population includes prematurely born very low birth-weight infants but, also, full-term newborns with significant congenital anomalies which will require extensive medical or surgical care. Therefore, the clinical focus embraces the development of infant organization and subsequent development over a long admission (months or years).

Infant organization relates to the 'integrated functioning between the infant's physiologic and behavioral systems' (D'Apolito 1991). While healthy newborns are equipped to handle the barrage of stimuli presented to them, pre-term and some compromised full-term infants may be unable to process the unpredictable input of the extrauterine environment. This lack of state organization causes distress in the infant, which may itself be difficult to resolve and is potentially harmful.

According to D'Apolito (1991), the distress is evident in disorganized physiological responses such as fluctuation in heart and respiratory rates that may result in apnoea or bradycardia, colour changes from pink to pale or dusky, increased stooling and inability to tolerate feeds, hiccups or sneezing, gagging or yawning and blood pressure instability.

Disorganized behavioural responses include frantic body movements and jitteriness, changes in muscle tone to flaccid or limp, an inability to modulate state, sudden state changes and/or prolongation of the alert state, limited use of self-consoling behaviours, inability to be consoled and an inability to habituate or decrease motor or state responses to noxious or repeated stimuli. These distress responses can be caused by simple care procedures such as turning the infant. Given the prevalence of handling and much more aversive stimuli, the infant can become distressed frequently and for extended periods each day. The theme of this chapter is to consider the role of music therapy for those infants for whom the neonatal intensive care environment and systems of care are detrimental in the development of infant organization and subsequent neurological development.

The inclusion of music therapy on the neonatal unit was instigated by the nursing team, who sought to provide more positive sensory experiences for those infants whose lives are dominated by invasive procedures and for those whose long admission means restricted opportunities for development. The underpinning philosophy, therefore, is that cautiously prepared and administered musical experiences can provide opportunities to allay the negative impact of extended admission in the neonatal unit. This is true for the infant but also for the primary carer (usually the mother) and other family members too.

The major part of this chapter will be completed through a case study which illuminates central aspects of music therapy for the post 30-week gestation infant. In this case the infant had a thoracic condition called Bronchopulmonary Dysplasia, which required a hospital admission of 13 months. The infant with Bronchopulmonary Dysplasia (BPD) offers an excellent example of how the simplest of musical experiences creates a potent developmental aid. The case presented here was my second referral for an infant with BPD and the longest relationship (spanning roughly 10 months).

Bronchopulmonary Dysplasia is 'a complex, multistage, structural and physiologic alteration of the lungs which occurs as a prolonged response to acute injury in the neonatal period'(Askin 1988, p.127). The combination of low birth weight, immaturity of the lung, oxygen therapy and mechanical ventilation are recognized as the primary factors contributing to the condition (Northway 1990). While it is common to see a lack of behavioural organization in premature infants, for infants with severe BPD this becomes more pervasive, effecting autonomic, visceral, motoric and state organization.

An American psychiatrist, Heidi Als (1992), has written extensively about the character and care of infants with BPD. She states that 'they present with a hypervigilant, pervasive state of panic and over-sensitivity to environmental stimuli such as lights, noises and especially touch' (p.345). Their inability to modulate their response to common sensory experiences causes chronic agitation. Methods typically used to interact, give care and console a pre-term infant appear ineffective and, at times, counter-productive. Social interaction and even gentle care giving may *increase* rather than reduce stress. Als notes that, for caregivers, the infant's behaviour appears to trigger feelings of resignation, helplessness and, often, outright anger. I have observed that nurturing may be abandoned and only physical care maintained.

Case example: Shaun

Use of recorded music

Shaun was born at 27 weeks gestation (13 weeks prematurely) and weighed 1050 grams. A large tumour in his left lung had been diagnosed antenatally and was surgically removed five days after his birth. The remainder of this lung was underdeveloped (less able to provide essential oxygen intake) and this, combined with complications of severe prematurity, resulted in BPD.

Shaun and his family were referred to me nearly 12 weeks after his birth for education on how music might be used to support Shaun's development. However, on my first visit, a member of his primary nursing team informed me that he was extremely irritable, becoming distressed very easily and remaining so over extended periods. This meant that he was using valuable energy and even more supplemental oxygen than was desirable. His mother, Crestina, agreed that transition to sleep was a distressing time for Shaun. Whilst the nurses understood the behavioural aspects of the condition, they were discouraged. They felt that the usual non-intrusive options such as swaddling, patting and even leaving him entirely alone were not working. Rather than introduce sedative medication, the primary nursing team asked me to programme some recorded music for him which would be available whenever it was needed.

I did not rush to intervene as Shaun presented with much more severe characteristics than the first BPD infant with whom I worked. The initial assessment included observation of behavioural systems organization based on the Als's synactive theory of development (1986). This theory proposes that development proceeds through the balancing of approach and yielding, resulting in integration of internal systems and organization of interactions with the environment. The observation documents a range of observable behaviours which indicate balanced, modulated functioning through to stressed and disorganized functioning. This provides a profile of behavioural strengths through to behavioural instability and fragility. I observed that, for Shaun, walking into his field of vision provoked jagged movements and speaking to him produced a tremor in his limbs or sometimes hiccups, both subtle cues of distress. If simultaneously touched or stroked, he grimaced and usually began crying. At this point his state of distress could not be modulated until many minutes after the stimuli were withdrawn. Shaun's inability to cope with the basic stimulation was overwhelming. He demonstrated no behaviours which indicated adaptation to the stimuli or regulation of response.

I realized that he did not need not more stimulation but regulation of the stimuli already present in his environment. Musical experiences needed to offer some insulation from noxious auditory stimuli and containment in support of organizing his responses to the world.

Before making decisions about the selection of recorded music, I met with Shaun's mother Crestina. Shaun's father was working and living in their home town more than three hours away. However, Crestina lived at the hospital throughout the admission. Crestina was very present in Shaun's day and took care of all Shaun's non-medical needs. She engaged him with the warmth and joy one sees in a mother with a healthy full-term baby. At first the professional team was suspicious that she was denying the severity of his status. However, the consistency of her behaviour eventually meant that we marvelled at her ability to remain joyous day after day. When I asked her about this positive outlook, she explained to me that she was his advocate in the world and that she helped to illuminate his true personality, which she sensed through his complex condition. She was a consistent and positive conduit between Shaun and the world.

Crestina's voice was an auditory beacon which Shaun tolerated. The nurses noted that he coped with her voice better than any other stimuli in his environment, giving further support to research findings on infant preference for maternal voice (DeCasper and Fifer 1980; Nöcker-Ribaupierre 1996). I felt uncertain about the potential of further female voices to offer him containment. I did not want to confuse him or dilute the potency of his mother's voice. Therefore, I proposed to Crestina that we use instrumental music and she agreed that it might provide a buffer from other environmental stimuli in the room. I believed that carefully selected instrumental music would mask some of the unpredictable elements of the environment and help him to retain homeostasis. With this support, we expected him to deal more ably with other stimuli, including his mother's unceasing love.

I prepared two audio tapes of 'sedative' music for the family's and nurses' use. Both contained music with sustained regular pulse, with little variation in timbre, dynamics, tempo and attack. The regular nature of this music offers an external regulation (Goldman 1991), supporting the infant's efforts to regulate himself. This principle has long been observed in the regulating and sedative effect of lullabies upon infants. Lullabies possess the recognized elements of repetitiveness, softness, simplicity, slow tempo and a 'soothing quality' (Trehub, Unyk and Trainor 1993). The intended purpose of lullabies is to help the infant make the transition in state from wake to sleep or distressed to calm. Thus the lullaby is used as the model for sedative music here.

The style of each tape varied a little, but reflected the parents' pre-existing stylistic preference for easy-listening popular music. Inclusion of parents' preferences is important at a number of levels. First, it gives support to the value of the family's life choices. There is a tremendous sense of grief and guilt in this early post-natal period (McHaffie 1990) and acknowledgement of even small life choices (such as music played during pregnancy) can be valuable. Second, I have observed that, given a choice of tapes, parents will generally choose and use more often the music with which they are familiar. Therefore, a selection of familiar or stylistically approachable music will ensure that the tapes are a more useful resource. At another level, it is vital that parents are able to nurture their infant. The normal methods of holding and cuddling or stroking and patting are often very restricted by the presence of equipment such as respirators or monitors on limbs and chest. Parents may feel powerless to support their infant in this environment. The small task of selecting and administering the music returns a small sense of control to the parent. Also, parents may be empowered to use their voices as an alternative nurturing source if sufficient auditory masking in the form of another auditory stimulus is present.

The first tape was an existing Australian-produced album called *Music for Dreaming*, a compilation of instrumental lullabies (e.g. Brahms's Lullaby, Hush-a-bye-Baby, Cradle Song, Golden Slumbers) produced with consideration of the US research on music therapy for infants. The second tape was a compilation of light orchestral pieces from the American company Windham Hill. These pieces include single-line acoustic instruments such as piano and guitar with small ensemble accompaniment from strings and woodwinds and some synthesizer accompaniment. This second tape was not used very much as the *Music for Dreaming* tape was more effective (see below).

The procedure for introducing recorded music to infants has become more rigorous now than at the time of this case study. As the potential of the music is more fully embraced in this context, the protocols are likewise developing to ensure its appropriate inclusion. At this time my initial instructions were given to the nursing team both in writing (in Shaun's file) and verbally to the nurse on duty. The instructions were to play the music only at times when Shaun appeared calm – that is, lying quietly alone or happily with his mother. The intention was to create a positive match between the stimulus and the behavioural state. Nurses verbally reported that the introduction of the music in quiet times lasted less than two days, after which they began to use the music at times when they were unable to soothe him to sleep in other ways. Fortunately, Shaun successfully tolerated the *Music for Dreaming* tape, and rapidly responded to it with desirable behaviours such as consoling and sleeping. As the main concern was for Shaun to conserve energy, sleep was pursued continuously through each day. Therefore, the tape was used each time the nurses hoped to settle him back to sleep (six to ten times per day).

Within three to four days of introducing the tapes, nurses began reporting Shaun's positive response to the music. I sought verbal feedback from the nurse on my arrival on the unit each day I attended the hospital. Their answers were general but definite. Several nurses referred to Shaun 'liking' the music. At the least, this meant that the music did not provoke the cues of distress which most stimuli did. At best, they noted that he attended to the music, distracting him from a general fussiness before it developed into distress. This allowed him the opportunity to fall asleep. It was also noted that if he was already distressed (crying, tremor, jagged movements) when the music was turned on, this behaviour still modulated and he settled. Crestina felt that he quickly came to recognize the music, moving his head and eyes to locate the tape player when it was turned on.

Previously, Crestina's voice was the only stimulus which promoted modulation of behaviour. However, after two weeks the consensus was that the recorded music was a reliable external regulator for Shaun, helping him to avert major distress. This responsiveness to external regulation was his first step to self-regulation later.

Use of multi-modal stimulation in the development of Shaun's voice

Face-to-face music therapy began when Shaun was 11 weeks corrected age (24 weeks after he was born) and finally able to achieve some regulation of his responses to the environment in which he lived. We decided on a period of more active intervention to promote the development of his positive vocal self-expression. I had observed that Shaun used little voice except to cry or protest. His voice was characterized by quite melodic intonation and his mother identified the potential for less adamant and more positive expression.

Shaun could still become distressed by sudden or new stimuli in his environment so I sought an introductory structure which would encourage acceptance of stimuli and active participation. Standley (1998) has developed a multi-modal stimulation protocol for use with infants as young as 32 weeks gestation to promote homeostasis and tolerance of stimuli. I felt that the initial stimulus of live singing would provide an excellent vehicle for promoting the musical qualities of Shaun's voice. Standley's protocol was adapted from the multi-modal sensory stimulation model by Burns *et al.* (1994), called the Auditory Tactile Visual Vestibular Intervention (ATVV).

The ATVV incorporates a programme of talking, stroking, eye-to-eye contact and vestibular motion. The initial stimulus here is spoken voice, with other stimulation added when the infant's observable signals indicate he is coping and discontinued when he is not. The decisions are made using a 'decision tree' which employs the individual's physiological and behavioural responses to determine a standard pathway of response from the carer. In Standley's (1998) adaptation, the initial stimulus is humming of the Brahms lullaby.

The protocols were relevant to Shaun as an older infant because they offered a straightforward method of controlling stimulation and supported my additional purpose of developing an active vocal response. However, the additional purpose required adaptations of the stimuli and the decision tree. In both the Burns and Standley protocols the base auditory stimulation of quiet talking or the humming of Brahms' lullaby supports a variety of tactile and vestibular stimulation. Because I sought to stimulate vocal response, I created variation in the auditory stimulus while maintaining a fairly static selection of tactile and vestibular stimulation.

This variable auditory stimulation needed to both affirm and stimulate Shaun's vocal attempts while retaining a sense of safety. I chose to improvise short melodic phrases which could invite his participation with ascending phrases and affirm his participation with slightly descending phrases. The choice of these melodic patterns was informed by the research of early communication development, which indicate that the melodic features of maternal voice convey communicative intention to the infant (Fernald 1989; Papoušek and Papoušek 1991).

Fernald (1989) suggests that the characteristic prosodic patterns of mothers' speech are meaningful to the pre-verbal infant. Papoušek and Papoušek (1991) analysed the intonation patterns of American and Chinese mothers to categorize the communicative intention of their utterances. They found that when communicating with their pre-verbal infant, mothers used the same melodic contours, despite the significant differences in the verbal language otherwise used. These 'universal' melodic contours included contour rises to encourage turn taking, imitation and evaluating infant state, and contour falls to soothe and reward for the infant's efforts. Thus, in the neonatal nursery, the contours of my improvised melodies sought to replicate natural maternal patterns and thus stimulate Shaun's natural responses.

Stylistically, I retained the consistency of the lullaby through the key elements of simplicity and repetition in the melodic phrases and lyrics (Trehub, Unyk and Trainor 1993). The improvised lyrics included frequent repetition of key words he had heard often, such as his name, and nurturing words, such as 'there, there, there'. The melodies were generally *legato* as *staccato* sometimes provoked a startle response. The dynamic ranged from *piano* to *mezzo piano* but, importantly, the sound was never whispered as it has been identified that the reinforcing value of the female voice is not present in whispering (Spence and Freeman 1996). The timbre evoked a 'loving tone' which Trainor (1996) identified as a recognizable aspect of infant-directed lullaby singing.

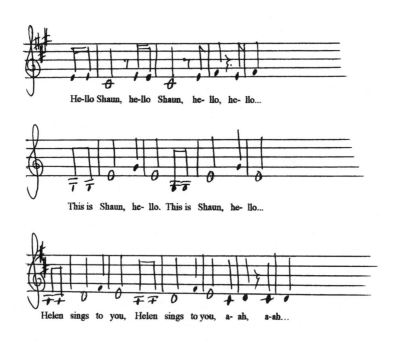

He-llo Shaun, he-llo Shaun, he- llo, he- llo...

This is Shaun, he- llo. This is Shaun, he- llo...

Helen sings to you, Helen sings to you, a- ah,   a-ah...

Figure 2.1 Samples of improvised melodies used to stimulate Shaun

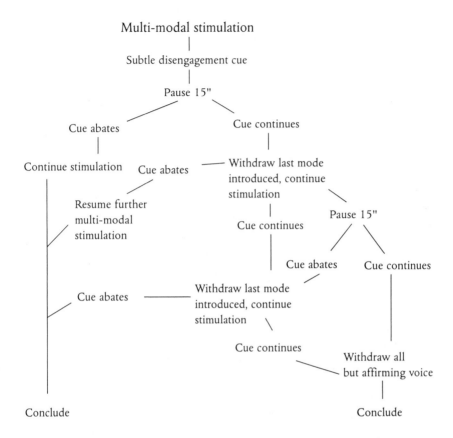

Figure 2.2 Decision tree, adapted by H. Shoemark from Burns, K., Cunningham, N., White-Traut, R., Silvestri, J. and Nelson, M. (1994) 'Infant stimulation: Modification of an intervention based on physiologic and behavioural cues.' Journal of Gynaecological and Neonatal Nursing 23, 7, 586.

I adapted the Burns *et al.* (1994) 'decision tree' (Figure 2.2), which enabled me to control the stimuli quickly and efficiently. The security of this protocol meant that Shaun's threshold for stimulation could often be reached but not easily crossed.

In Shaun's case this meant that on observing disengagement behaviours such as yawning, hiccuping or facial grimace, I halted the stimulation for 15 seconds. If the disengagement cue abated, the stimulation was recommenced; if it did not abate, the stimulation was continued but without the last sensory mode or vocal variation. If the disengagement cue escalated, the protocol was quickly reduced to the most acceptable stimulation level and then discontinued for the day.

Outcomes for the multi-modal stimulation

The benefits of the decision tree were immediate, particularly in the earliest phase of face-to-face work. The pause in stimuli, or removal of the last stimulus added, ensured that he gained much successful rehearsal in dealing with stimulation near his threshold whilst minimizing distress.

In the early sessions Shaun attended to the initial stimulus of my sung voice with calm interest. I used a predominance of soothing descending melodic phrases, using his name as the main lyric. He occasionally responded with very brief *pianissimo* utterances such as 'uh' or 'erh'. In the second session I introduced the visual stimulation of eye contact as he sought the direct interaction. He responded with appropriate patterns of fixed gaze and gaze aversion – that is, modulating how much visual stimuli he was taking in. He also began to vocalize, using some descending melodic lines in response to my ascending melodic 'invitations'.

When I also introduced the stimulation of holding him in session six, he responded with only a few very brief utterances before rapidly disengaging (yawns, followed by facial grimaces). In keeping with the protocol, I withdrew the last stimulus of holding him (returning him to his cot) and, once he had settled, I recommenced with the auditory and visual stimuli, which he tolerated again. In further sessions I seated him in an infant chair in his cot (so we were face-to-face), where he was then able to engage with me using eye contact, facial expressions, some touch on the hands and a developing array of vocalizations. Our 'dialogues' built from moments in these early sessions to several minutes at the conclusion of the programme (some eight weeks later).

In terms of the stimulus itself, I felt that the maintenance of repetition in the melodic phrases was particularly useful in providing recognizable motifs for the opening and closing of the protocol. I also favoured these motifs as soothing responses to disengagement cues which continued or escalated.

The use of short melodic phrases was productive. While I was singing I could observe Shaun's impending response and quickly conclude any phrase to allow him space to sing. My shortness of phrases reflected his short phrases, offering some equality in the vocal relationship. In time I was able to subtly increase the musical complexity of the stimulus without compromising this relationship. He enjoyed the sounds he made and often repeated them with variation in the intensity or duration. He thus developed an awareness of my patterns of affirmation and invitation, and successfully used them himself with clear communicative intent.

The initial character which had pervaded Shaun's voice quickly blossomed in this safe context. He soon initiated his new-found positive vocal interplay with other significant people in his world, thus evoking positive vocal responses from them and creating new possibilities for communication.

My role for the remainder of his admission decreased as he became more able to engage with the world around him. I continued to provide recorded music, which is still used at home for sleep and rest times.

In an environment where even momentary random or unfamiliar sounds can be harmful, I regularly use the protocol as a precautionary measure in my first contact with infants. I use it regularly with other infants with BPD and it has proved effective in quickly modulating stimulation to suit their individual requirements.

Discussion and conclusion

Use of recorded music

In my experience, hospitalized infants generally respond to recorded music in a positive manner. It seems that music is perceived as an acceptable experience by even the most immature infant (Cassidy and Standley 1995). The predictable quality of the programmed music quickly becomes familiar and positive associations build, making music a reliable strategy for soothing a calming infants.

Since this case study, more recent practice includes observational assessment of all referred pre-36-week gestation infants for tolerance of pre-recorded music and live singing. Infants are behaviourally assessed and, where monitoring is already occurring, physiological impact is assessed. Where pre-recorded music is to be used, and is determined to be a safe stimulus, verbal and written instructions are given to nursing staff and parents to use on demand – that is, where the nurse or parent feels a soothing stimulus would be advantageous, music may be used. We recommend that it is not played continuously to avoid possible habituation and loss of potency. After this, the role of the music therapist is to evaluate the efficacy of the recorded music and extend the selection of tapes as appropriate.

The analysis of presentation modes by Cassidy and Ditty (1998) is helpful in clarifying benefits and considerations. At the Royal Children's Hospital, modes include predominantly free-field cassette players and occasional use of adult earphones laid beside the infant's head. Determining factors include the economic rationalization of new equipment versus existing free-field cassette players and the intrusiveness of the mode for the infant. As these infants are already restricted and distressed by life-supporting and monitoring equipment, it is undesirable to add to this with ear cups, phonopad earphones or earmuffs. The volume of free-field music must be checked near the infant's head to ensure a suitable quality of sound is available to the infant while not intruding into the auditory environment of other infants.

There is a clear need for research about the value and application of recorded music for the older pre-term infant. Quantitative data is difficult to collect because of the diverse variables involved in the treatment and progress of these infants. A series of case studies may illuminate best practices for this complex group.

Live singing as a developmental stimulus

To sing for hospitalized infants demands that the music therapist fully realizes the breadth of his/her vocal ability. The therapist can exercise immediate and subtle control over the voice, perhaps more so than any other instrument. This is significant when there is the possibility of causing real distress to the infant if unsuitable stimulation occurs.

In presenting the sung voice as an intervention for hospitalized infants, the music therapist must, at any moment, choose the musical elements to be featured or restricted. I believe that the therapist's intuitive selection of elements in that moment is supported by extensive training and experience in controlling the elements for music performance. Likewise, a functional knowledge of music theory informs the successful stylistic marriage of musical elements in creating forms such as the lullaby. This theoretical understanding will enable the music therapist to adapt infant-oriented forms such as the lullaby for maximum benefit. The lullaby can be used in its entirety (Standley 1998) as an effective unimodal stimulus when working with pre-32-week gestation infants who are beginning to tolerate stimulation, or the discriminate use of the recognizable elements of the lullaby (Trehub, Unyk and Trainor 1993) can preserve the reassuring aspect of this form as a basis for further interaction – as with Shaun.

While modern medicine enables infants as small as 22 weeks to physically live outside the womb, we have much more to learn about sustaining a quality of life in these tiny infants. When the initial medical crises have passed, many infants remain in the hospital environment for extended periods. Their quality of life is undeniably poor, as the life-saving equipment and procedures, at the least, confine life experiences and, at worst, provoke pain and distress. The long-term impact of this first hospitalization is now being realized in reduced functioning and subsequent services for older surviving children (Standley 1998).

The inclusion of music therapy services acknowledges the need to address the whole child in this first admission. The interventions described here clearly need research to empirically establish efficacy. Of primary importance is the need to establish assessment, administration and evaluation protocols to ensure consistency of application.

Acknowledgements
My thanks to Shaun and his parents Crestina and Phil for their support in preparing the case study.

Glossary

Apnoea: absence of automatic breathing.

Bradycardia: abnormal slowing of heart rate.

Congenital anomalies: any defect present at birth; may be inherited, occur during pregnancy or during childbirth.

Homeostasis: relatively constant state in the body, naturally maintained.

References

Als, H. (1986) 'Synactive model of neonatal behavioural organization: Framework for the assessment and support of the neurobehavioural development of the premature infant and his parents in the environment of the neonatal intensive care unit.' In J.K. Sweeney (ed.) *The High-Risk Neonate: Developmental Therapy Perspectives.* New York: The Haworth Press.

Als, H. (1992) 'Individualized, family-focused developmental care for the very low birth-weight preterm infant in the NICU.' In S. Friedman and M. Sigman (eds) *The Psychological Development of Low-Birth Weight Children.* Annual advances in applied developmental psychology. Vol 6. Norwood, NJ: Ablex Publishing Corp.

Askin, F. (1988) 'Pulmonary disorders in the neonate infant and child.' In W. Thurlbeck (ed.) *Pathology of the Lung.* New York: Thieme Medical Publishers.

Burke, M., Walsh, J., Oehler, J. and Gingras, J. (1995) 'Music therapy following suctioning: Four case studies.' *Neonatal Network, 14,* 7, 41–49.

Burns, K., Cunningham, N., White-Traut, R., Silvestri, J. and Nelson, M. (1994) 'Infant stimulation: Modification of an intervention based on physiologic and behavioural cues.' *Journal of Gynaecological and Neonatal Nursing 23,* 7, 581–589.

Caine, J. (1992) 'The effects of music on the selected stress behaviours, weight, caloric and formula intake, and length of hospital stay of premature and low birth weight neonates in a newborn intensive care unit.' *Journal of Music Therapy 28,* 4, 180–192.

Cassidy, J. and Ditty, K. (1998) 'Presentation of aural stimuli to newborns and premature infants: An audiological perspective.' *Journal of Music Therapy 35,* 2, 70–87.

Cassidy, J. and Standley, J. (1995) 'The effect of music listening on physiological responses of premature infants in the NICU.' *Journal of Music Therapy 32,* 4, 208–227.

D'Apolito, K. (1991) 'What is an organized infant?' *Neonatal Network 10,* 1, 23–29.

DeCasper, A. and Fifer, W. (1980) 'Of human bonding: Newborns prefer their mothers' voices.' *Science 208,* 1174–1176.

Fernald, A. (1989) 'Intonation and communicative intent in mothers' speech to infants: Is the melody the message?' *Child Development 60,* 1497–1510.

Goldman, J. (1991) 'Sonic entrainment.' In D. Campbell (ed.) *Music Physicians for Times to Come.* Wheaton, Ill.: Quest Books.

Kaminski, J. and Hall, W. (1996) 'The effect of soothing music on neonatal behavioural states in the hospital newborn nursery.' *Neonatal Network 15,* 1, 45–54.

McHaffie, H. (1990) 'Mothers of very low birthweight babies: how do they adjust?' *Journal of Advanced Nursing 15,* 6–11.

Nöcker-Ribaupierre, M. (1996) *Music Therapy and Premature Birth.* Paper to the World Congress in Music Therapy, Hamburg, Germany.

Northway, W. (1990) 'Bronchopulmonary dysplasia: Then and now.' *Archives of Disease in Childhood 65,* 1076–1081.

Papoušek, M. and Papoušek, H. (1991) 'The meaning of melodies in motherese in tone and stress languages.' *Infant Behavior and Development 14,* 4, 415–440.

Spence, M. and Freeman, M. (1996) 'Newborn infants prefer the maternal low-pass filtered voice, but not the maternal whispered voice.' *Infant Behavior and Development 19,* 199–212.

Standley, J. (1991) 'The role of music in pacification/stimulation of premature infants with low birthweights.' *Music Therapy Perspectives 9,* 19–25.

Standley, J. (1998) 'The effect of multi-modal stimulation on developmental responses of premature infants in neonatal intensive care.' *Pediatric Nursing.*

Standley, J. and Moore, R. (1995) 'Therapeutic effects of music and mother's voice on premature infants.' *Pediatric Nursing 21,* 6, 509–512, 574.

Trainor, L. (1996) 'Infant preference for infant-directed versus noninfant-directed playsongs and lullabies.' *Infant Behavior and Development, 19,* 83–92.

Trehub, S., Unyk, A. and Trainor, L. (1993) 'Adults identify infant-directed music across cultures.' *Infant Behavior and Development, 16,* 2, 193–212.

CHAPTER 3

Premature Birth and Music Therapy

Monika Nöcker-Ribaupierre

Music therapy and premature birth is an area of work which is quite new in clinical practice, for music therapists as well as for physicians in newborn intensive care units. Because of the technical progress of intensive medicine, infants at an ever earlier stage of development have a chance to survive. In addition to many other problems, the difficult psychological situation of child and mother is attracting increasing attention. In addition to other efforts, auditory stimulation with the mother's voice is being integrated into regular activities in some hospital units since it has generally been found to be very effective.

I have developed this application of music therapy on an interdisciplinary basis by combining hermeneutic and statistical empiricism. It is an integrative music therapy area of work which is situated between the functional and the psychotherapeutic aspects of music therapy.

After an introduction regarding life in intensive care units and the physical conditions for acoustical stimulation in very low birth-weight infants, I will describe my study, the method, the results and its philosophy, including the influences of other related disciplines, and give some comments for its clinical application.

Introduction

Because of the overwhelming presence of technical instruments, the light and the constant level of noise, with frequent disruptive alarm signals, it is difficult to see the patient in all the different types of intensive care units as an individual. In these surroundings we find patients with no possibility of communicating in the way people normally do. We can only observe their state of consciousness and development according to electroencephalographs

(EEGs), heart rate variations, oxygenation saturation, audit of reflexes, level of agitation and vegetative reactions. These are patients whose vital functions concerning growth, survival or prolongation of life have to be maintained through intensive medicine.

When using music as a therapeutic medium to mask the noise, or to reduce adverse stress reactions or find a pathway to his or her soul, we are only able to describe whether this acoustic medium reaches the patient, not how it affects him/her emotionally. It is possible to see signs of stress, anxiety and discomfort while watching the patient and evaluate his/her status through measurable physiological effects. The patients in intensive care units must often be medicated to reduce stress and its associated physiological manifestations. This stress may also be exacerbated by the routine of treatment, the light exposure and the excess noise in these units.

Music, recognized as a means of decreasing or alleviating these signs, has been used throughout the last decade in many health care settings – such as coronary care, surgery, anaesthesia, post-anaesthesia recovery and intensive care units (Davis-Rollans and Cunningham 1987; Moss 1988; Spintge and Droh,1988). The positive effects of music have been evaluated (Munro 1978).

Like adult patients, neonates also seem to react adversely to their new life in this stressful unphysiological environment. First, I would like to give an impression of the acoustic environment that premature babies are exposed to during their stay in newborn intensive care unit(s) (NICU). The general noise in NICU is about 55–65 dB, within the incubator today about 56–62 dB. (For comparison, the normal background noise in an office is at a level of about 60 dB.) The noise in the lower frequency range, below 500 Hz, such as from machines and human voices, reaches the baby unfiltered. Frequencies above 500 Hz hardly penetrate the incubator. Nevertheless, conversations in front of the incubator have an intensity of up to 90 dB inside the incubator and impulse noise (e.g. putting something on the incubator, slamming the door or the telephone) up to 114 dB. The latter two causes are greatly influenced by the attitude of the staff (Wolke and Eldridge 1991).

Very small premature infants react from the beginning to these unphysiological, incalculable outside noises visibly and measurably with adverse reactions. These are reflected in sleep disturbance, restlessness and crying (often inaudibly because of the tube, but visibly), decreased oxygen saturation and heart rate levels, so-called apnoeas and bradycardias, wide fluctuations in blood pressure and increased agitation and restlessness that means acceleration of heart beat and breathing.

During the first two weeks the children are often startled so badly that they have to be sedated, because anxiety has a negative effect on respiration and circulation. After this period they do not react anymore to such disturbances. This behaviour is regarded as 'getting used to' or 'conditioning', in the medical sense a positive effect. Since the early 1990s the therapeutical use of music in intensive care units for patients who are not accessible to verbalization is increasing, especially in the adult units.

The basis for the indication of music therapy for patients who are not accessible to verbalization, such as comatose or so-called apallic patients and premature infants in intensive care units can be explained within the phylogenesis of hearing development. In contrast to other sensorical systems, the auditive system has a first integration centre in the brainstem (medulla), in the colliculus inferior. This centre has links with motoric and pre-motoric centres and also via the thalamus with the limbic system. In phylogenesis the cortical system is post-connected to this old and complex system. This means that the impact of the colliculus inferior on the limbic system is largely independent of the cortical involvement. According to this finding, there should exist a direct route of acoustical impact which is independent of the cortex and which directs vegetative as well as emotional and motivational manners of behaviour (Groth 1995).

This way is preserved, even in cases of severe injury to the cortex. It is already functioning before the cortex is fully developed – in the ontogenesis, the child is developed a long time before birth to take in acoustic impressions. At the age of 18 weeks the hearing system is structurally and functionally developed to the point where it can function (Rubel 1984). It is possible to observe, via ultrasound, reactions to acoustically evoked signals in the unborn child after 24 weeks of gestation (Birnholtz and Benaceraff 1983) and in the premature child after 26 weeks of gestation (Nöcker, Güntner and Riegel 1987).

Prenatal acoustic impressions and post-natal ability to discriminate

The foetus lives intrauterine within an acoustic environment which is characterized by biological sounds – that is, the heartbeat and visceral sounds. In addition, the child is exposed to many acoustic influences which also have a psychologically formative character. During pregnancy the continuous acoustic experience, the starting point for the relationship of rhythm and human being, is the heartbeat of the mother.

The basis for the relationship between human beings through the environment, communication and speech is created by the mother's voice. For therapeutic work it is not so much the discursive but the presentative content of the voice. Essential and formative for the psychological effect are sound, melody and rhythm of the voice.

The developing child is able to store and to remember acoustical impressions during his prenatal time and, post-natally, to distinguish them from new, unknown impressions.

This has been observed, especially in the United States, in numerous studies with newborn babies (DeCasper and Fifer 1980; Fernald 1982; Standley and Madsen 1990). All these studies addressed the question of whether newborns could remember sounds they had heard before birth and whether they have preferences for certain voices. Measurements were made using different parameters, such as behaviour and oxygen content in arteries.

These studies have shown that newborn infants can distinguish the words they had heard repeatedly during their prenatal life from unfamiliar words (DeCasper and Fifer 1980), that they prefer female voices to male voices and the mother's voice to other women's voices (DeCasper and Fifer 1980; Standley 1990) and that they can distinguish an ascending intonation from a descending one if both scales are sung by the same voice on the same vowel (Fernald 1982).

As these studies verified, the capability to perceive acoustically is determined genetically – that is, it exists before birth and during the time the premature baby has to stay in the incubator in order to survive.

Developmental follow-up studies show delay and difficulties in the future life of these very low birth-weight children, which indicates the necessity to improve psychosocial treatment. Research, especially from the United States, has shown that a variety of stimulation techniques may help the pre-term infant to overcome some of the adverse neurological effects and negative consequences of pre-term birth and prolonged hospitalization. For this reason, many multimodal and purely acoustical stimulation programmes have been carried out. Isolated music stimulation – such as the lullaby by Brahms, mother's voice, lullaby-type singing, female vocal sounds or music on the basis of womb sounds and heartbeat – have shown particularly effective and significant results, such as reducing observed stress behaviour and pacification (Busnel, Mosser and Relier 1986; Caine 1991), significant increase of oxygen saturation levels (Caine 1991), significant increase of oxygen saturation levels and decreased levels of agitation (Cassidy and Standley 1995; Collins and Kuck 1991; Standley and Moore 1995), increasing weight gain (Caine 1991; Chapman 1979), stronger positive effects on female infants than on male infants in increasing weight gain (Coleman *et al.* 1998), length of hospitalization (Caine, 1991) and significant earlier discharge (3–5 days) from the hospital (Coleman *et al.*1998). According to the health programme in the United States, it is an objective of all these studies to develop the role of music therapy as an effective area within prevention and stimulation programmes.

Significance of premature birth

Due to the continuous improvement of the technical aspects of intensive medical care during the last 20 years, it is possible for less and less mature babies to survive.

Today the limit is 23–24-week term babies and a birth weight of about 500g. That means survival at a stage of development at which all sensory organs have sufficiently grown and developed to receive sensory impulses – survival in a non-physiological surrounding, characterized by necessary intensive medical over-stimulation, the mental and emotional deficit, and endless painful experiences. These very little infants spend about two months in the incubators and, on average, four months in the hospital.

I have worked for many years as a music therapist in a newborn intensive care unit (NICU), where I developed the idea of providing these babies with acoustic impressions different from the noise of the technical machines surrounding them. First, we thought of masking the technical noise level and stimulating vital functions by exposing infants to the music of Mozart and the mother's voice – following the theoretical basis of the Tomatis Method.

But in my practical work I discovered that most of the mothers considered it very strange to play music for their baby but they were all very happy to talk on a tape for their baby. It became quite obvious that, especially at the beginning of this extreme situation, the mothers find it very difficult to establish a relationship with their baby.

In this process it became necessary for me to look for theoretical thoughts from related disciplines, such as medicine, developmental psychology, new analytical and bonding theories, and infant research, to understand what happens in the situation of a premature birth. I put together relevant interdisciplinary findings to explain the conditions for a stimulation programme which takes into account both the infant and his/her mother.

So I regard my music therapy approach as psychotherapeutic because I am oriented on the process and development of relationship and bonding as a fundamental basis of life and on the psychological significance of the prenatal acoustic experience of the musical parameters in a mother's voice. Despite this orientation, I had to research and evaluate my stimulation method mainly in a quantitative way in order to be accepted and understood in intensive care units.

But before describing the study, I first have to give some comments on the theoretical basis.

The importance of bonding

In terms of the development of the mother–infant bonding, premature birth means that an infant and a mother are separated from each other at the wrong time. Through this break of the psychophysical continuum, they miss out on the experience of an important time of being together.

The mother is physically weakened and also finds herself psychologically in an isolated state of mind. She is not able emotionally to understand the situation. She does not see or feel her baby to be a separated person. In identification with her baby she regards herself as the cause of anxiety in an overwhelming technical environment. Additionally burdening are feelings of guilt, lacking self-worth, the separation and the fear for her baby's survival. All these feelings make it most difficult for her to develop into a primarily positive relationship with her baby.

In my approach to the subject of premature birth I start from the assumption that during this early period of bonding one has to regard, and to treat therapeutically, mother and infant as a unit. Therefore, when considering ways to accompany their development therapeutically, it is necessary to take into account the situation of both of them.

A music therapy-oriented stimulation programme with the mother's voice as a medium is able to achieve this. I have been thinking about what kind of basis for living and experience this voice can convey to the infant.

My auditory stimulation combines two different approaches: the functional therapeutic approach of retaining or replacing something lost and a music therapy approach which addresses the developing subjective experience within the relationship between mother and child.

This means that auditive stimulation, due to its qualities of creating relationships, is able to help both to build bridges from the intrauterine life through the time in NICU to life at home. Therefore, auditive stimulation enables an independent intrapsychological activity towards a renewed relationship between mother and infant.

The therapeutic situation

In the psychoanalytic treatment of adult patients, messages and dreams often emerge which are interpreted as memories of the earliest time of life. Since the 1940s this has led a number of psychoanalysts (Fedor-Feyberg 1987; Graber 1974; Hau and Schindler 1982; Schindler and Zimprich 1983) and representatives of prenatal psychology (Ammon 1982; Graber 1974; Janus 1990) to assume the existence of prenatal experience. They conclude from this that various psychological disturbances have their cause in the prenatal period.

But trying to understand the psychodynamics of prenatal life or to reconstruct the experience of premature infants on this basis is, I believe, subject to the danger of adultomorphism. Therefore, I searched for any theories that tried to explain the understanding of the emergence of traces of memory within the self of the child.

On this point, Daniel Stern (1985) has made some fundamental statements. Based on the observation data in infant research, he concludes that the infant does have a subjective experience. Thus he creates a connection between empirical infant research and psychoanalysis. He describes the emergent self-worth as a primary, organizing and structuring principle which already controls the earliest development. In contrast to psychoanalytic theory, Stern offers the hypothesis of a holistic development principle which, from the beginning, includes other significant persons.

In other words, the psychological regulation of life occurs through exchange of social behaviour, the interaction between the child and his/her mother or parents. In this context the different ways of feeling, which accompany all elementary events of life, play the decisive role. Stern describes them as 'vitality affects'. He explains them as follows:

> Abstract dance and music are examples *par excellence* of the expressiveness of vitality affects. Dance reveals to the viewer-listener multiple vitality affects and their variations, without resorting to plot or categorial affect signals from which the vitality affects can be derived. The

choreographer is most often trying to express a way of feeling, not a specific content of feeling. (p.56)

And, later:

Like dance for the adult, the social world experience by the infant is primarily one of vitality-affects before it is a world of formal acts. (p.57)

From the very beginning of his life, the infant demonstrates many abilities which allow him to connect his different social and cognitive experiences. These abilities are genetically determined. They either exist at birth or they can develop later, provided the neurological development conditions and the environment are right.

If the infant is not able to bring together the early traces of memories, disturbances occur during this time and one can expect that the body-soul development may take on pathological forms. Then it is possible that birth before the regular time requires archaic psychological forms of defence to enable psychological survival, such as autistic and psychotic splits.

Premature birth and music therapy

What can a therapeutic support be like when it takes into account both persons, the mother and the infant?

At the beginning of this process the mother should be empowered to respond with activity to the feeling of helplessness. This is achieved by helping the mother to give something of herself through body contact. Often, the opportunities for tactile stimulation, such as touching, holding, cuddling or 'kangarooing', are very limited during a period of many weeks.

Therefore, it is only logical to suggest that the mother reaches out for her infant through another sensory channel, the acoustic one. She can talk to her baby, give him a name, tell him something of herself. She can imagine that her baby is able to listen to her and that they both have a common space of experience, like the 'intermediary space' of Winnicott (1965), in which both share in listening to what she is conveying to him.

The mother's voice is something alive, through which vitality affects are conveyed to the infant in this disembodied world of the incubator. The manner in which the mother moves and acts, her whole personality which is familiar to the foetus, is also reflected in her voice.

During the prenatal period the mother's voice is an element of connection. She is bodily close, and at the same time contains the whole concept of verbal communication – which, in terms of development psychology, takes place at a later stage. At this stage what is important is not the word but the vocal expression, with its musical parameters according to the early state of the infant's development. At the same time, this vocal expression guarantees the continuity of prenatal and post-natal life.

Birth ahead of the regular time means, for the baby, the beginning of a difficult, life-threatening time in a disembodied environment, characterized by unprotectedness and pain, with little connection to what is understood as life – connection to a human being. For it is only through a relationship and interaction that a child becomes able to survive mentally.

There is a very impressive example of this theme when Emperor Frederick II was looking for the primeval language of mankind. He experimented on a number of newborn babies who were well looked after. But without verbal interaction or caring physical contact they all died.

The premature newborn infant lacks all the stimulation emanating from his mother's womb: acoustic experiences, warmth, body contact, bio-chemical exchange – all aspects of an early emotional and social communication.

When accompanying the infant therapeutically it is necessary to give something to him that can be a way to a connection with his mother – her voice, non-verbal emotions and musical content of her voice. This does not refer to the significance of this voice as the basis for developing speech but to the creative mental impact of the voice – through its sound, melody and rhythm which each infant will recognize – to carry or to continue the prenatal emotional interaction.

Rhythm and sound convey the beginnings of early childhood experience, as does the rhythm and sound of the mother's voice. Feelings of the mother are transmitted to her infant through the musical parameters of her voice.

I was able to observe this in the reactions of two children during an early period of my work. Both infants had been born with life-threatening medical problems after 28 weeks' gestation. Both mothers suffered mentally and were full of fear and incapable of talking to their baby. When standing at the incubator, both readily accepted my suggestion to tape their voices, for playback to the infants. But their voices were noticeably weak, flat and depressive. At the age of 34 weeks both infants began to cry when the taped voice was played but not when the mothers were talking directly to them. In the meantime the mothers' voices had changed to a brighter, more powerful sound because of the improved conditions. After a new tape was made, both infants reacted immediately with head turning and looking to the source of the new sound.

Another important issue is the infant's ability to react to acoustic influences. From the outset, very small premature infants react to the disembodied, unpredictable outside noises in the unit, visibly and measurably, with psychophysiological disturbances. After a period of about two weeks they no longer react to such disturbances. This behaviour is regarded as becoming conditioned to the sounds or habituating to them. But, according to my observations, there is no conditioning to the mother's voice, even after playing the same tape for a period of several weeks. Unless they are sick and/or have been sedated or are asleep, they react to this voice with full attention.

Eagle (1988) addresses the different theories of the development of object relationship. He says:

> that all results suggest that the interest in objects as well as the development of feelings of attention are not... the result of having other needs satisfied, but that they are a decisive independent aspect, which is the expression of a congenital desire to establish cognitive and affective ties to objects in the world. (p.18)

From the very beginning, tactile and kinaesthetic stimulation is the decisive dimension to which the infant reacts. In this context an infant's selective preferences for certain stimulative figurations are autonomous congenital affections that could already be observed immediately after birth.

What Eagle describes with respect to the tactile and kinaesthetic stimulation I will expand through the subject of auditive stimulation. Since the hearing organ is developed so early in the ontogenesis, I assume that, next to the neurological development significance of acoustic stimulation, the mother's voice during pregnancy plays an important role in the development of intrapsychological representations for the beginning of bonding. From that I conclude that during the time of intensive medical care after premature birth it is possible, with the help of the mother's voice, to open a psychological space for the child – that is, a space where development happens.

Full-term infants, immediately after birth, show the ability 'to recognize an object with the help of one sense (touching), which they had got to know through another sense (seeing)' (Eagle 1988, p.30). A full-term, two-day-old infant is able to recognize and distinguish a dummy from a different looking one which he got to know only by sucking.

This developmental step may already take place several weeks prior to full-term birth, as from around 36 weeks onwards the premature infant cannot be pacified any longer through his mother's voice from the tape alone but only through a combination of acoustic and tactile stimulation like caressing, holding or being carried.

Auditory stimulation with the mother's voice – a description of the method and its results

After a pilot study with high and normal frequency ranges of acoustic stimuli following the Tomatis Method, I started my research programme with the mother's voice.

The focus of this study was primarily to examine the effect of the mother's voice on physical activity and the transcutaneously measured arterial oxygen tension ($tcPO_2$) of very low birth-weight infants. It also set out to find out if this outcome could possibly influence the development of the child in connection with the behaviour and stabilization of the mother.

The mothers of all the infants were interviewed. I explained the study and asked them if they would agree to my programme. After this interview the mother talked on a tape.

At this point I have to say something about the recording. At the beginning of the study I thought that a mother should sing – for example lullaby-type singing – and I suggested that she try it. But it was obvious that in this extremely isolated situation it was impossible for a mother to sing normally – during all these years I have met only two mothers, out of more than 200, who were able to sing. Very often it was even impossible to freely talk, so I used to propose reading – for example, *The Little Prince* by Antoine de Saint-Exupéry. The infant heard this recording through a small loudspeaker in the incubator five or six times a day, for half an hour at a time, at about 65 dB, preferably starting in the second week of life, but certainly as soon as clinical stabilization was reached, and continued until about the 36th week post-menstrual age (PMA). Experience has shown that at this time the infant gets fidgety because it expects a person, not only a voice. The stimulation time was regulated with a timer in order to establish consistency of the intervention on a day-to-day basis and, with consideration of care episodes, to avoid any disturbances, and because of the character formation of early stimulation the infant should not learn to associate its mother's voice with treatment procedures.

During the first observation study I examined (with the help of two medical students) the direct effect of the mother's voice on the child by measuring the physical activity (Prechtl Score) and the transcutaneously measured arterial oxygen tension (tcPO$_2$). Subjects were nine very low birth weight oxygenated infants (gestational age 26–29 weeks, birth-weight 780–1270g). The children were their own control: they were observed one day with and one day without stimulation during a period of mean 8.2 weeks. As a whole this study showed: (1) The infants react visibly and measurably to the mother's voice after the age of 26 weeks PMA if they are not shielded off through illness or medication and (2) The mother's voice has a physically calming effect on the infant, resulting in a significant decrease of activity and a significant increase of tcPO$_2$. Whether and to what extent this significant calming effect of auditory stimulation influences the development of the children was the main question of the second study.

For this study I compared the development of 24 stimulated infants (gestational age 24–30 weeks, birth weight 650–1270g) with 24 conventionally treated infants. The latter were randomly selected but matched for sex, birth weight (+/-100g) and gestational age at Munich clinics. The duration of the stimulation was at least six weeks. These infants were subjects of the prospective observational study by Riegel, Ohrt and Wolke, 1995) at the same time. All infants in this study passed a detailed investigation by release and the following assessments: at the corrected age of five and twenty months and at 4.8 and 6 years by using special assessment scales.

The baseline parameters on the clinical state of both groups were not different. By comparing development, data analysis showed that at the corrected age of five months the stimulated infants showed significant advanced motor and verbal development (Griffiths Scales, p<.05). This trend's was still present at the corrected age of 20 months, though insignificant. At six years of age the verbal activities as measured with 18/18 infants (Heidelberger Sprachentwicklungstest (HSET) and Kaufmann (K-ABC)) showed an improvement in the stimulated infants, in one part significant (HSET:VS p<.05).

Because of the small number of cases, one can regard this only as a tendency. But this tendency provides an important indication for the significance of early auditory stimulation and the psychological stabilization of the mothers that comes with it. For this last evaluation I had three items:

1. Data analysis showed that the mothers of the stimulated infants breastfed significantly more often (50% versus 12.5%) and longer (one year versus three months).

2. Using non-informed observers for group comparison at the five-month assessment, these mothers were also seen to be less burdened and physically more stable. This outcome could have an impact on the development of the child.

3. Personal statements – after discharge I asked the mothers to write a statement about their experience with the recording of her voice and the accompaniment that went with it. All mothers regarded this recording to be very supportive for their infants and their own stabilization.

Mother's voice, the therapeutic medium

There are, as mentioned before, a variety of stimulation programmes with music, especially with lullabies. Because of their global cultural qualities due to uniformity of melody, rhythm and performance (Papoušek 1994), lullabies may also be particularly suitable to help premature babies to recover. The last study, by Coleman *et al.* (1998), showed positive physiologic and behavioural effects of male and female voices singing lullabies to premature babies.

But, because of my different way of regarding prematurity, in my approach music cannot be the therapeutic medium. Music, in this case mainly lullabies, is proven to be helpful to soothe the baby and to have positive effects on his physical well-being and development in many ways but it does not help to increase the disturbed bonding process or to decrease psychological problems that could follow a too early separation. Also, the symbolic value of music, which plays such a decisive role in therapy with adult patients, makes no sense when the patient still lives in a pre-conscious, pre-symbolic world.

I use the mother's voice as the medium because the mother's voice, for the infant, is a substitute for her physical presence, but, at the same time, it is a symbol for the relationship.

At the beginning of life rhythm and sound do not yet have any cognitive symbolic qualities. The premature infant is not yet sufficiently developed to be able to symbolize. This is because the formation of symbols occurs on the basis of the creation of inner representations, requiring the presence of consciousness and memory.

Rhythm and sound accompany the beginning of early childhood experiences – in addition, I submit that they also create relationships if they are mediated through the mother's voice. After a premature separation of the physical connection between mother and infant, that took place many weeks too early, it is possible to preserve for the infant, with the help of the musical parameters of his/her mother's voice, a continuum of primary acoustic representations for the development of the infant's subjective experience. So auditory stimulation is a receptive music therapy method for the premature infant and is also a psychotherapeutic form of crisis intervention for the mother.

As mentioned before, the event of a premature birth means, in addition to the crisis of anxiety, devastation to self-esteem and feelings of guilt, a severe narcissistic indignity. This situation makes it difficult for the mother to develop a pathway to her baby, which is very different to that which she had in mind. It happens in my practical work that the mother's behaviour changes immediately when she gets the opportunity to do something for her baby, to think about what she can tell him/her.

While talking, her voice allows her to be separated from the infant. At this moment she does not have to create a 'We' because the infant is becoming an object who becomes separated from the damage of her narcissistic feeling. Later, when a nurse tells her of the infant's reactions – the calming down, becoming attentive, sometimes smiling or falling asleep while hearing her voice – she knows that her baby will get to know her in spite of the separation and that it has responded to her offer of a relationship. As a result, she visits more frequently and stays longer. She has discovered her own potential. This is an important condition for resuming the interrupted bonding process.

Discussion

The auditory stimulation provided by the mother's voice combines two different approaches: the functional therapeutic approach of retaining or replacing something lost and influencing adverse reactions to intensive care; and a music therapy approach which addresses the developing subjective experience within the relationship between mother and infant, the bonding process.

The mother's voice is something alive, through which vitality affects are conveyed to the infant in the technical world of the incubator. The manner in which the mother moves and acts, her whole personality (which is familiar to the foetus), is also reflected in her voice.

During the prenatal period the mother's voice is a point of connection. It is physically close and contains, at the same time, the whole concept of verbal communication, which, in terms of development psychology, takes place at a later stage.

One can say that auditory stimulation enables an independent intra-psychological activity towards a renewed relationship between mother and infant. The therapeutic quality of the musical and emotional content of the mother's voice is, due to its qualities of creating relationships, able to help both mother and infant to build bridges from the intrauterine life through the time in NICU to life at home.

Clinical application

Over the last ten years interdisciplinary follow-up studies to examine the effect of early intervention and/or educational intervention on the health and development of the very low birth-weight infant have been carried out. They were all begun during the hospital stay of the infant and continued after discharge from the hospital. Besides the different aspects of the baby's functioning, these interventions also focused on the interaction of mother/parents and infant and on encouraging and supporting the mother's knowledge and confidence.

All these studies, such as the Vermont Intervention Program (Achenbach and Rauh 1988), and the Infant Mental Health Program (Blair, Ramey and Hardin 1995; Brooks-Gunn, Liaw and Klebanov 1992, 1994; McCarton et al. 1997; McCorminck et al. 1993), came to the conclusion that, medically and developmentally, very low birth-weight infants benefit significantly from individualized and environmental care which also pays attention to the parent–infant bonding and the parent–infant interaction.

As mentioned before, the emerging literature shows that the developmental aspect is now, and will continue to be, the topic of interest in intervention programmes for very low birth weight infants.

But none of these studies have paid attention to music therapy until now. The previously mentioned music therapy studies in the United States and also my study had been evaluated separately and have only recently been integrated into multidisciplinary programmes or medical treatment (Standley 1998).

Although both music therapy methods have been proven to be significantly helpful in terms of development and have started to be integrated in intensive care units in the United States and Germany, hospitals have been reluctant to assign positions for this work. It depends largely on the music therapist's personal commitment and persuasiveness whether he or she is allowed to work in a NICU.

I think that, on the basis of the described findings, it is helpful to work in NICUs by combining the two aspects, starting with the therapeutic use of the mother's voice to support the interrupted bonding process and, later, of lullaby-type music, following the studies from the United States. A programme like this could take into account the special medical and developmental situation of the individual infant as well as the social and psychological situation of the mother/parents. This treatment should start in the intensive care unit and should continue into early childhood.

The role of the music therapist is to support the mother and to help her work on developing her resources to cope with this extreme situation, with focus on the interrupted bonding process and the developing mother–infant interaction as the basis of development.

Guidelines for practice

Recording

Select a quiet and undisturbed place without any outside or technical disturbances. Be careful with the microphone while recording. Use an endless tape or a similar CD where you can repeat the recording. For the text select a story or fairy tale, but preferably use free talking or lullaby-type singing.

Note: the recording is only for the infant, no one else will listen to it. So please leave the mother alone while she is talking. You must remember to allow time for the mother to become used to the microphone.

The recording should be made as soon as possible, in any case as soon as clinical stabilization is reached. But take care of the feelings of the mother.

For the incubator

Put the recorder in a place where it doesn't disturb the day-to-day clinical treatment and put the external loudspeaker into the incubator. You need a timer to determine the playing times. This should not coincide with the caretaking procedures (ask the nurses). The times should be arranged with the mother (possibly five or six times a day for 15 to 30 minutes each – that depends on the infant and the mother's presence, and should be related to normal time, between 7 p.m. and 9 a.m.). Fix the volume with the help of the mother, no louder than just masking the incubator noise. Watch the infant! Repeat the recording after three weeks.

First, record only the mother (because of feelings, bonding process, etc.) and later, if wanted, add the father. Watch the infant! Because of the state of development at about 36 weeks, the infant may get fidgety with the tape alone. Once that happens, remove the loudspeaker (tell the mother ahead of time). Find out if there are additional possibilities of help – social worker, verbal psychotherapy, self-help groups, etc.

Glossary

Adultomorphism: regarding something from the adult point of view.

Apallic patient: patient who lost main cerebral functions.

Apnoe (apnoic episode): episode of cessation of breathing for at least 15 seconds.

Bradycardia: episode of slowing down of heart rate below 60 beats/min.

Developmental tests:

1. *Griffiths's Scales:* test for examination of the infant's functional development at 5 and 20 months.

2. *HSET (Heidelberg Speech Developmental Test):* test to examine speech development (active/passive and understanding).

3. *Kaufman K-ABC (Kaufman Assessment Battery for Children):* test to examine cognitive development (intelligence and information processing).

Kangarooing: carrying baby with skin-to-skin contact.

NICU: newborn intensive care unit

Premature baby: born before 36 completed weeks of gestation.

PMA: post-menstrual age.

tcPO$_2$: arterial oxygen tension, measured transcutaneously.

Tomatis Method: a training for listening intended to condition the practice of listening on the basis of the significance of intrauterine listening, developed by Alfred A. Tomatis (French physician).

References

Achenbach,T.M., Howell M.S., Aoki, M.F., Rauh, V.A. (1993) 'Nine-year outcome of the Vermont Intervention Program for low birth weight infants.' *Pediatrics 91,* 1, 45–55.

Ammon, G. (1982) 'Zur Psychosomatik von Frühgeburt und psychosomatischer Erkrankung.' In T.F. Hau and S. Schindler: *Pränatale und Perinatale Psychosomatik.* Stuttgart: Hippokrates.

Birnholtz, J.C. and Benaceraff, B.R. (1983) 'The development of human fetal hearing.' *Science 222,* 516.

Blair, C., Ramey, C.T. and Hardin, M. (1995) 'Early intervention for low birth weight premature infants: Participation and intellectual development.' *Am Ass on Ment Retard, 99,* 5, 542–554.

Brooks-Gunn, J., Liaw, F. and Klebanov, P.K. (1992) 'Effects of early intervention on cognitive function of lbw preterm infants.' *Journal of Pediatrics 120,* 3, 350–359.

Brooks-Gunn, J., McCarton, C.M., Casey, P.H., McCormick, M.C., Bauer, C.R., Bernbaum, J.C., Tyson, J., Swanson, M., Bennett, F.C., Scott, D.T., Tonascia, J. and Meinert, C.L. (1994) 'Early intervention in low-birth-weight premature infants.' *JAMA 26,* 272, 16, 1257–1262.

Busnel, M.C., Mosser, Ch. and Relier, J.P. (1986) 'Preliminary results on the effect of acoustic stimulations on premature infants.' *Pediatric Research 20,* 1056.

Caine, J. (1991) 'The effect of music on the selected stress behaviors, weight, caloric and formula intake, and length of hospital stay of premature and low birth weight neonates in a newborn intensive care unit.' *Journal of Music Therapy 28,* 4, 180–192.

Cassidy, J.W. and Standley, J. (1995) 'The effect of music listening on physiological responses of premature infants in the NICU.' *Journal of Music Therapy 32,* 4, 208–227.

Chapman, J.S. (1979) 'Influence of varied stimuli on development of motor patterns in the premature infant.' In G. Anderson and B. Raff (eds) *Newborn Behavioral Organization: Nurs Res Impl.* New York: Alan Liss.

Coleman, J.M., Pratt, R.R., Stoddard, R.A., Gerstmann, D.R. and Abel, H.H. (1998) 'The effects of male and female singing and speaking voices on selected behavioral and physiological measures of premature infants in the intensive care unit.' *International Journal of Arts Med 5,* 2, 4–11.

Collins, S.K. and Kuck, K. (1991) 'Music therapy in the neonatal intensive care unit.' *Neonatal Network 9,* 6, 23–26.

Davis-Rollans, C. and Cunningham, S.G. (1987) 'Physiologic responses of coronary care patients to select music.' *Heart and Lung 16,* 4, 370–378.

DeCasper, A.F. and Fifer, W.P. (1980) 'Of human bonding: Newborn's prefer their mother's voices.' *Science 208,* 1174–1176.

Eagle, M.N. (1988) Neuere Entwicklungen in der Psychoanalyse: eine kritische Würdigung. Internat Psychoanalyse München Wien.

Fernald, A. (1982) *Acoustic Determinants of Infant Preferences for 'Motherese'*. Unpublished doctorate dissertation, University of Oregon.

Fedor-Feyberg, P.G. (1987) *Pränatale und Perinatale Psychologie und Medizin*. Saphir Älsvjö, Schweden.

Graber, G. (ed) (1974) *Pränatale Psychologie*. München: Kindler.

Groth, B. (1995) Evolution der akustischen Kommunikation. Congress Munich, communication.

Hau, T.F. and Schindler, S. (eds) (1982) *Pränatale und Perinatale Psychosomatik*. Stuttgart: Hippokrates.

Janus, L. (1990) *Die Psychoanalyse der Vorgeburtlichen Lebenszeit und der Geburt*. Pfaffenweiler: Centaurus.

McCarton, C.M., Brooks-Gunn, J., Wallace, I.F., Bauer, C.R., Bennett, F.C., Bernbaum, J.C., Broyles, R.S., Casey, P.H., McCormick, M.C., Scott, D.T., Tyson, J., Tonascia, J., and Meinert, C.L. (1997) 'Results at age 8 years of early intervention for low-birth-weight premature infants.' *JAMA 8*, 277, 2, 126–132.

McCorminck, M.C., McCarton, C., Tonascia, J. and Brooks-Gunn, J. (1993) 'Early educational intervention for vlbw infants: Result from the Infant Health and Development Program.' *The Journal of Pediatrics 10*, 1993, 527–533.

Moss, A. (1988) 'Music and the surgical patient: The effect of music on anxiety.' *Association of Operating Room Nursing Journal 48*, 1, 64–69.

Munro, S. (1978) 'Music therapy in palliative care.' *Can Med Ass J 119*, 1029–1034.

Nöcker, M., Güntner, M. and Riegel, K.P. (1987) 'The effect of the mother's voice on the physical activity and the tcPO$_2$ of very premature infants.' *Pediatric Research 22*, 221.

Papoušek, H. (1994) 'The origins of musicality.' In C. Faienza (ed) *Music, Speech and the Developing Brain*. Milano: Guerini.

Riegel, K.P., Ohrt, B. and Wolke, D. (1995). *Die Entwicklung Gefährdet Geborener Kinder bis zum Fünften Lebensjahr*. Stuttgart: Enke.

Rubel, E.W. (1984) 'Ontogeny of auditory system function.' *Ann Rev Physiol 46*, 213.

Schindler, S., Zimprich, H. (eds)(1983) *Ökologie der Perinatalzeit*. Stuttgart: Hippokrates.

Spintge, R., and Droh, R.(1988) 'Ergonomic approach to treatment of patient's postoperative stress.' *Can J of Anesthesia*, 5, 1988, 104–106.

Standley, J.M. (1998) 'The effect of contingent music to increase non-nutrive sucking of premature infants.' ISMM Melbourne 1998, communication.

Standley, J.M., Madsen, C.K. (1990) 'Comparison of infant preferences and responses to auditory stimuli: Music, mother and other female voice.' *Journal of Music Therapy*, XXVII 2, 54–97.

Standley, J.M. and Moore, R. (1995) 'Therapeutic effects of music and mother's voice on premature infants.' *Pediatric Nursing 1*, 2, 90–95.

Stern, D.N. (1985) *The Interpersonal World of the Infant*. US: Basic Books Inc.

Winnicott, D.W. (1965) *The Maturational Processes and the Facilitating Environment*. London: The Hogarth Press.

Wolke, D. and Eldridge, T. (1991) 'Environmental care.' In A.G.M. Campbell and T. McIntosh (eds) *Forfar and Arneil's Testbook of Pediatrics*. Edinburgh: Churchill Livingstone.

PART TWO

Developmental Disability

CHAPTER 4

Contact in Music

The Analysis of Musical Behaviour in Children with Communication Disorder and Pervasive Developmental Disability for Differential Diagnosis

Tony Wigram

It is often difficult for music therapists to explain in words exactly what happens in music therapy sessions and there is diversity in the profession between more structured styles of work and the more dynamic and psychotherapeutic approaches. The easiest way to understand what is occurring in music therapy in the tradition with which I am most familiar and work within is that it involves the development of a shared musical experience between the client and the therapist. This musical experience incorporates the development of a relationship with the client where the music that is created represents not only the personality and mood of both the client and the therapist but also unconscious feelings and thoughts which will emerge. The client must feel very free and secure in the session and develop their own confidence in being able to express themselves musically (through instruments and vocally) without any required musical skill or experience. The role of the therapist is to create a musical framework within which the client can function and to develop through that framework a relationship with the client where they are able, together, to gain an insight into the client's inner life. The use of improvised music is frequently the medium for creating this music dialogue with a client and has formed the basis of many approaches and traditions (Alvin 1965, 1975, 1978; Bruscia 1987, 1991; Bunt 1994; Heal and Wigram 1994; John 1995; Nordoff and Robbins 1971, 1975, 1977; Odell-Miller 1995; Pavlicevic 1995, 1997;

Priestley 1975, 1995; Wigram 1991a, 1992a, 1997; Wigram, Saperston and West 1995).

In previous publications in the field of assessment through music therapy, particularly in assessing communication disorders in children, I have referred more generally to the structure of sessions, but mainly from the point of view of what objective criteria one uses, giving some examples to illustrate the general purpose of assessment (Wigram 1991b, 1992b, 1995a, 1997). Defining a method of working in music therapy is a risky proposition as it is frequently open to criticism and question, yet I have taught a 'method' to students and therapists in order to give a framework for assessment. In order to contextualize the process of music therapy as a tool for diagnostic assessment, it is necessary to describe the framework within which I work.

Structure and flexibility in music therapy assessment

Coming from therapeutic influences which range from Client-Centred Therapy (Raskin and Rogers 1989) and Cognitive Therapy (Beck and Weishaar 1989), I do not subscribe to a totally free structure in music therapy and often use 'play rules' or 'givens'. My starting point when embarking on therapy with clients can be defined more clearly through an assessment period in which I will try to understand the needs of my clients and formulate some focus on the aims and purpose of therapy. I use music in a structured and unstructured way through improvisation, alternating between a directive and non-directive approach as may be appropriate to the needs of the client. I also believe in a flexible approach, accepting all sounds to be within a therapeutic context, without necessarily requiring a musical framework which may over-structure the client.

Music therapy as a diagnostic tool for assessing communication disorder and autism

Music therapy can play a very significant role in the assessment process with children who have communication disorders, because of the non-verbal nature of the medium when working with pre-verbal communication systems. A music therapy framework allows children a potential for revealing pre-verbal and alternate communication systems that they have developed, which can, in turn, support or negate a diagnosis of autism and point in a different direction. Normal babies are biologically primed to play an active role in social interaction and they have an inherent sense of timing that controls 'turn-taking dialogues' with others. This is very important in the music therapy process as the nature of music making between two people relies on timing and turn taking – sharing and creating that is the essence of communication. Trevarthen *et al.* (1996) describe the early development of mother–baby interaction, the relevance of timing and facial recognition, and the interpretation and response to emotion in facial expressions particularly well in the context of the emerging difficulties of autistic children.

When looking at the difficulties an autistic child emerges with from babyhood, one can see that the handicap of a brain dysfunction interferes both with the coding and also the making sense of 'messages' (for example, spoken language, facial expression, etc.) and with the use and understanding of timing. Therefore, a baby with autism receives messages that they are confused by and, as a consequence, retreats from social interaction. In an effort to develop communicative interaction with their baby, parents and others will continue to send messages, usually quite directly, whereupon the baby with autism begins to develop 'cutting-out' mechanisms which can be gaze avoidance and stereotyped motor movements. These, in turn, can develop into obsessions and rituals which the baby with autism develops in an attempt to ground themselves in a familiar and secure structure in an otherwise chaotic and confusing world. They don't develop the normal pre-verbal 'conversational exchange' that is typical with normal babies and, therefore, don't move on into normal social interactions or the formation of social relationships – which, in its turn, leads into normal language development. In history taking we frequently find the absence of normal pre-verbal 'babble', which is expressive and meaningful at a pre-verbal level and is inflected and formulated in phrases. This babble is timed 'turn-taking' exchanges between the parents and the baby. The intoned sounds which babies use to express needs and feelings from about nine months onwards are inbuilt and inherent, not learned. In this way a baby attracts attention, expresses emotion and engages in social exchange. Music making in an improvised and free way, both with instruments and also with vocal sounds, is a way of revisiting this early phase of communicational exchange using simple rules and free, unlearnt sounds. The children who are assessed in music therapy at Harper House can readily demonstrate a capacity for going into this medium for demonstrating their desire to communicate, where verbal language for one reason or another – due to either pathological or social disabilities – has not properly developed.

Information seeking in the therapy assessment

A therapy assessment session is different from a regular therapy session. In diagnostic assessment the therapist has to take responsibility for a number of different factors:

- exploring the child's range of responses
- exploring the child's lack of response
- looking at both the potential of the child and their difficulties
- evaluating the child's response to the novelty of the situation
- testing a diagnostic hypothesis proposed for the assessment
- evaluating the child's response in terms of their general potential
- evaluating the child's response in terms of their potential to benefit from music therapy
- evaluating the child's response in terms of their potential for responding to other forms of therapy or intervention
- considering the child's behaviour and response in a music therapy assessment in relation to the wider picture of the child's response to other media.

I am conscious, when undertaking a therapy assessment, particularly for diagnostic purposes, that during the process of the session I work at different levels using different approaches. However, this is not a situation where I jump from one idea to the next and the session remains essentially a therapy session where a subtle movement from one framework or scenario to another is necessary to sustain and develop a therapeutic relationship, and sustain the engagement and confidence of the child.

I am particularly interested in looking at the child's response to subtle variations in approach and framework. If a child is easily engaged, and enjoys close contact, I will at some point in the session establish a distance from the child and retreat from the engagement to see what happens. If the child is more responsive to structure and finds that approach easier, I introduce a period of very free activity without rules or direction. At times I will use conventional and repertoire music, comparing this with their response to improvised music. While at times allowing the child the freedom to control what is happening in the session, at other times I will make demands on the child to explore their reaction when under a certain amount of pressure or when they are required to participate in something to which they might demonstrate some resistance. In this particular area a careful balance needs to be maintained, where one can go so far with a child to explore their resistance but not too far to create a potentially disturbing or damaging effect. Because we are frequently assessing children with communication disorder, I include in the session both verbal and gestural cues and look for any evidence of abnormal or unusual responses to sound, hyperacousis, pseudo-hyperacousis or hair-trigger reactions.

The music therapist has at his disposal a wide range of instruments that children can use in therapy sessions. In a conventional therapy session children will often choose favoured instruments or instruments to which they feel most connected, and these may remain the instruments they use for the whole of the session. In an assessment therapy session I am interested to explore their reaction to using a wide range of instruments and I would feel that I had failed to gain an overview of the child's potential if they spent the whole session using exclusively one or two instruments.

Finally, in a therapy assessment session I am focusing on differentiating autistic disorders from others and am particularly interested in developing strategies for sharing and turn-taking in music making, and in the use of the instruments. When children begin to explore instruments and learn how to make music creatively, they normally use the instruments appropriately, either from having seen how to by modelling or instinctively. The way of playing is to create music intentionally that is expressive and has musical intentionality. I have found some recurring patterns in the way some autistic children use musical instruments and create musical sounds that can separate them from children with communication disorder or other forms of learning disability:

Physical and tactile behaviour:

Flicking and twiddling – that is, with drum sticks, small instruments.

Spinning – tambours, cymbals, rotary drums, jingles on a tambourine.

Fiddling – that is, with parts of an instrument, with the nut in the middle of the cymbal.

Playing with instruments tactilely but without musical intention – turning tambourines back and forth, bunching the bars on the windchimes, plucking the strings of a guitar individually and watching the vibration.

Choosing instruments for their material quality – that is, being more interested in metal instruments.

Pathological elements in musical material:

Establishing routines that don't change in the way of playing.

Lining up instruments.

Using instruments to play sounds in order – for example, perseverative and repetitive scale playing on the piano, xylophone, metallophone, etc.

Sequencing – for example, making an unchanging rhythmic sequence or playing a beat consecutively on a drum, cymbal, chair and the floor, and repeating the sequence.

Social interaction and communication elements in music making:

Children on the autistic continuum reveal significant difficulties in:

| Turn-taking | Sharing | Anticipating |
| Reflecting | Copying | Empathic playing |

Because of their lack of interest and awareness of others, they can also show a lack of interest and ability for responding to or sharing changes in tempo, rhythm, timbre, intensity and many other elements of a shared musical engagement.

I am not proposing that *all* autistic children reveal these difficulties in assessment *or* that they cannot develop abilities and motivation for these elements in interpersonal engagement in music. What needs to be clear is that an analysis of musical events and the meaning or interpretation of the child's music must be considered in terms of intentionality and meaning to either express themselves individually, initiate a connection to the therapist or respond to music initiated by the therapist.

Aspects of this process, and the process of the session which I have described above, will be illustrated in a case example.

Assessing communication disordered children – a model structure for sessions

I have found, through working in a child assessment and diagnostic unit, that one needs to find a balance between developing a therapeutic relationship and seeking out relevant information which may be important to specifically posed diagnostic questions.

This session structure is quite flexible and I do not always follow this procedure with every child. However, I do try to work through a process with the children where I am mixing both free, undirected, elements of the session with more structured and focused areas.

As I am frequently trying to evaluate the pathological origin of a communication disability, such as autism, the equipment chosen for use in the session is quite deliberate. What I will now describe is a flexible sequence of events that occur roughly in the order defined but are not all necessarily present in every assessment and can vary depending on how the process develops.

Opening

- ∘ Free exploration
- ∘ Supportive improvisation
- ∘ Waiting time/revealing time.

I allow the child to begin the session, when entering the room, by waiting to see what instrument they might choose straight away or whether they wander around looking at the instruments or ignoring them. After a short time, I frequently go to the piano and play, quite unintrusively and supportively, some gentle improvised music. I try to allow my intuition into the client's way of being to generate 'empathic improvisation', a method described by Alvin (Bruscia 1987) where the therapist attempts to reflect their feeling of the client's physical and emotional state in their music – giving a musical interpretation to the client of how the therapist sees and feels them.

I try not to make any demands 'musically' or require any response from them at this time. This is a waiting time, a time to watch and see what they do, whether they choose to relate to me or whether they choose to ignore me. It is also a time to see what they choose to use in the room and what they ignore.

Free improvisation

- ∘ Tonal and atonal
- ∘ Reflective and mood responsive.

While they are exploring the instruments, or, alternatively, while they are waiting to see what might happen next, I will try to match their mood musically. I reflect back to them the feeling I am receiving from them, the mood they are in and, perhaps, to some extent, the mood I am in at the beginning of this session.

Structured improvisation

- Therapist on piano, client on 'chosen' instrument
- Emerging turn-taking and sharing strategies
- Musical 'questions and demands', both rhythmic and melodic
- Matching and non-matching styles.

After the free improvisation period I will try to focus the client more on the particular instrument they have chosen to use predominantly. I will initially work from the piano and try to initiate and develop turn-taking with the child, and then, subsequently, see how they respond if I share the instrument they are using or make a dialogue with them on a similar or complimentary instrument.

Musically, I initiate 'questions and demands', rhythmically and melodically. The purpose here is to begin to structure the musical dialogue we may have developed by helping the child with some musical frameworks, such as simple rhythms, melodies and phrases of melodies, to see what they pick up and how they respond. Also, it is a provocation to which they may make an alternative musical statement or response, or which they may resist.

I will frequently match, mirror or reflect their musical material, or, alternately, provide opposite ideas to the musical material they are producing.

This is a significant part of the session as it involves a relationship-building process through music, which some children will accept and some will reject.

Introduction to new instruments

- Windchimes, metallophone, gong
- Varying styles: game playing, sharing, discussing, free improvisation, repertoire.

When the attention or interest of the child begins to decay to the structured improvisation session on their chosen instrument, I will, at this point in the session, introduce new instruments. I am quite specifically choosing the three instruments mentioned above – they are all metal; they can develop a different experience for the child; they are all interesting diverse shapes and produce sustained sounds.

With the windchimes I often develop 'game playing' with the children, peering through the bars at them, enjoying tactile experiences with the instrument and seeing whether they intuitively use them with musical intention or for a more tactile experience.

With the metallophone I can explore their intuitive skill in knowing how to play this instrument and also whether they introduce scale playing and alternate hand playing.

Finally, the gong is an instrument we can both share the experience of playing and which usually provokes a very excited reaction from some children, and, possibly, a frightened reaction from other children. I can empathize with the frightened reaction by reacting in a startled way to loud sounds they may make on the instrument. This is another mechanism for developing sharing and turn taking.

Working through the free improvisation section, the structured improvisation section and this section with new instruments, I am at all times able to experience the personality of the child in their music making. Unconscious and hidden moods, anxieties, emotions and resistances will emerge throughout this period of time.

Discussing

By this time in the session, if it is appropriate and if I have not already initiated discussion, I will start to introduce more verbal material (depending on the verbal skills and understanding of the client), asking them questions about what they are doing, what they like and what they would like me to do.

I also introduce repertoire, if it is appropriate. Sometimes, the parents mention that their children have favourite songs, television programme themes, cassette tapes, etc., and I sometimes work with this material from the piano while they are playing or singing.

Pausing

- Waiting time.

At this point I will frequently pause and, sometimes, even 'switch off' or move into the background. I am interested to see whether the child takes the initiative to move on to a new idea, return to a favourite instrument, want to go back upstairs to their family, or some other direction, or simply demand more attention from me. It is a period of transition, a time to reflect on what we have done and look for a new direction in the session.

Containing

- Continue on favourite instrument
- Look at attention span
- Playing to child
- Pretend play, role play.

Various things can happen at this time. We may return to the child's favourite instrument and re-establish some work with that. I may take some time to play to the child at this point, especially if they have begun to lose their capacity to sustain their own direction. I may also introduce some structured activities at this point, such as pretend play or role play, where I may give the instruments characters, such as 'Daddy drum', 'Mummy drum' and 'Baby drum', and see if we can enact some musical dialogue which will give an insight into the child's experience of family dynamics. In evaluating a potential diagnosis of autism, this is also a musical equivalent to exploring imaginary play. I may also become more structured and directive at this point and introduce some rhythm-matching experiences with the child where I play certain rhythms and ask them to play rhythms back to me.

Some of what goes on at this time is an evaluation of the child's ability to sustain their own attention, as well as their ability to respond to my attempts to contain and sustain their attention.

It is a containing time, containing the child within a space, keeping the child near to me, keeping the child focused on the instruments and on the music we are making together.

Sustaining

- Amplified microphone
- Sound bubble
- Guitar.

The final section of the session before we close is frequently towards the end of the child's attention span and interest, and I introduce some new experiences for the child. I have an amplified microphone for vocal improvisation to see if the child can understand how to make sounds that come out through the speaker or whether the child will listen to me making sounds. It is a time to explore vocal exchange, if it has not already happened, and find out if the child will say some words, or sing, either freely in an improvised way or a song they may know.

I also introduce the 'sound bubble' at this time, which is an electronic instrument produced by the firm 'Toys for the Handicapped' that makes a variety of different sounds, depending on which of the touch-sensitive buttons you press. This activity helps evaluate their response to physical contact as the sound bubble can be used to create sound by touching parts of the body while completing a circuit.

By this time, the child may still sustain their interest in what is happening or may start to reject any new developments.

Closure

 ◦ Saying goodbye to instruments
 ◦ Saying goodbye to room.

I try always to close the session by taking the child round to say goodbye to the instruments that they have used, as a way of stopping the session. Then we say goodbye to the room before we go back upstairs to where their parents have been watching the session.

This is an important part of the session, particularly if the child has either become distressed for any reason or has started to develop strong resistance to what we are doing. It is a moment at the end to have a final sharing together of the experiences we have had and I either encourage the child to go round and touch the instruments or make one or two final sounds on them as a way of saying goodbye.

I have defined the elements in these sessions and put the process into the order in which these events quite frequently occur. However, this order sometimes varies and, although I try to include most of these events to gain a full picture of the person engaged within these various frameworks, it is always necessary to respect the boundaries and needs of the client.

Analysis and interpretation of musical material

When presenting the results of a music therapy assessment or a period of music therapy, the documentation of musical material, and the analysis of the musical experience that has been present during the session/sessions with children, is, I believe, fundamental and necessary. While there are many models for evaluating music therapy in the literature, very few involve a detailed analysis of musical material, and the documentation of changes or sameness in the musical material, to provide supportive evidence of change or lack of change in the music therapy process. In case material in the literature one frequently encounters clear descriptions of behavioural change in clients, with quite vague references to musical events that have led to the interpretations of change. This does not in any way invalidate the interpretation that has been made and I am not questioning the therapeutic judgement that has been offered of the benefit of music therapy in facilitating change, development, improvement or insight. However, it is unclear to other music therapists, and even more unclear to other professionals, on what basis interpretations were made when there is a lack of description using musical parameters of the musical behaviour which indicated the change described.

One assessment procedure that focuses specifically on musical elements as the basis for analysing change or lack of change in clients are the Improvisation Assessment Profile(s) (IAPs) (Bruscia 1987). For the last three years I have been employing the IAPs to analyse the musical material in diagnostic assessment sessions with children who have come to Harper House. Despite the fact that the IAPs have been in the literature for some years, my understanding is that there is quite a limited use of this assessment method currently. They have been translated into Norwegian (Stige and Ostegaard 1993) and have been used in Scandinavia. However, they are a complex, detailed and extensive method of analysis and this complexity can be off-putting to the practitioner where, when using the IAPs in their most comprehensive way, a short excerpt from a music therapy session could take several hours of analysis.

I have selected two of these six profiles as most relevant for diagnostic assessment of communication disorder and modified and adapted the procedure to be usable at a practical level.

In the complete set of profiles Bruscia has defined six specific areas of investigation: autonomy, variability, integration, salience, tension and congruence. Each profile provides specific criteria for analysing improvisation and the criteria for all the profiles form a 'continuum of five gradients or levels, ranging from one extreme or polarity to its opposite' (Bruscia 1987, p.406).

The two profiles that I have chosen to use most frequently for the analysis of musical material with children who have communication disorder are autonomy and variability. Described below are the profiles and scales for autonomy and variability.

Case study: Barry

Barry was a child of five years and one month who was referred to the Harper House Children's Service for assessment and diagnosis. He was described as being strangely withdrawn with odd traits. At three-and-a-half years old he walked on his toes and did not speak intelligibly. He spoke his first word at 18 months and started babbling and intonation patterns at two years. In his early history he was reported to have had very little real development in his language, apart from his ability to echo back what he had heard. He was reported to enjoy playing with cars but lining them up in rows. His symbolic play was developing but rather concrete and quite primitive. By report from the speech and language therapist, he initiated very little himself as far as social interaction was concerned and his speech and language skills were reported to be more close to that of a two to two-and-a-half-year-old child. He was displaying evidence of ritualistic behaviour and could become quite frustrated at times with tantrums when he didn't get what he wanted. At the first appointment Barry appeared to make no spontaneous social contact and had a rather blank stare with very little smiling or interested expressions. Previous paediatric assessment had concluded that it was quite likely that Barry was autistic, although it was also hypothesized that he might be a child with a learning disability and a very severe language disorder which might have led to him demonstrating autistic types of behaviour.

Before discussing the way Barry responded in the music therapy assessment, and describing the three sections that I analysed using the IAPs, it is interesting to look at the way Barry was responding in the Speech and Language Therapy (SALT) assessment and the art therapy assessment. The SALT assessment was a structured, directed session to explore Barry's potential for both verbal and non-verbal communication. It was noticeable from the beginning that Barry had quite a strong will and his main interest in the box of items the speech and language therapist was working with from the floor was the toy train. After completing an inset puzzle he spontaneously tried to get to the box and take out the train. Despite the therapist's attempts to engage him using a puppet doll and a musical toy, Barry continued to leave the table and try to get into the box. She allowed him to use the train on the table. What he then did with it was also interesting: he took it in his right hand and swept it from side to side on the table. When the therapist took it from him and pushed it towards him, attempting to initiate a sharing of this toy and non-verbally encouraging him to push it back to her by holding out her hands, he merely reverted to rolling the train from side to side.

Looking at the art therapy session, the therapist modelled drawing and painting for him on the paper and Barry was quite effective in copying, to a fairly exact degree, what the therapist was doing. When the therapist drew a line across the bottom of the page, Barry copied it. When the therapist drew a line up the side of the page, Barry copied it to the point of standing up and leaning over so his line could reach exactly the same point as the therapist's. When the therapist drew squares and began to fill them in, Barry quickly got the idea and also filled in squares that the therapist provided on the paper. However, given freedom to do what he wanted to do, and provided with paintbrushes and a palette of seven or eight different coloured paints, Barry began to draw from side to side on the paper, putting one colour on top of another until there was a thick coat of paint streaked with different colours going from side to side. The pattern looked quite similar to the train and one can conclude from this that, without structure, Barry's creative play is quite limited. He didn't use the paints in any way specifically to create figures or pictures but indiscriminately drew from side to side with many different colours until there was a lack of differentiation in the colour and it was a dirty grey, black mess.

Music therapy assessment

There were three clear sections that I selected from the music therapy session to analyse:

Section 1: a 6–7 minute excerpt where Barry played the rotary timpani drum, timp-tom drum, snare drum and cymbal, while I played the piano. Included in this section was also a vocal exchange.

Section 2: Barry was playing the metallophone and, sporadically, the cymbal, while I was accompanying him on the piano.

Section 3: Barry and I were playing one piano together.

Section 1

In this opening section Barry started by experimenting to find out the sounds of the different drums in front of him and the cymbal. I offered him different sticks that he could use and he chose the hard-headed drumsticks. He began with a regular pulsed beat and I supported him on the piano with a gradually accelerating, tonal and chordal/melodic improvisation. After a few seconds I paused on a tremolo octave in both hands, a transitional technique, waiting to see if he wanted to continue with a pulsed beat. His playing slowed down as he became uncertain and he made single beats on the cymbal and the snare drum either side of the rotary timpani that he was playing. Already, he had demonstrated variability in the instruments he was using on the variability profile, events which I was charting as timbre variability. He continued to play in a pulsed beat, but it began to vary in speed significantly and there was clear evidence of follower, leader and partner activity going on that I could score on the autonomy scale in terms of tempo. He initiated accelerando and I followed, subsequently initiating my own accelerando. He became excited, squealing and quickening his beat.

We built up to a climax, which he chose to stop suddenly, turning and hitting the cymbal with a single beat. This was one of a number of events where he demonstrated initiative and, therefore, leadership in the musical interaction and sequence. After a short 10- to 15-second experiment with both the cymbal and the snare drum, he reverted back to the rotary timpani, reintroducing the pulsed beat, which I followed. I continued to lead him melodically and he watched and followed my playing quite carefully both in tempo and volume. For a moment he began to set up a pattern of beats, going from the cymbal to the timpani to the snare drum, in the sequence similar to what he had been doing in the art therapy session and the speech and language therapy session when he was making a side-to-side movement. This only lasted for a short period, as he began to follow again my lead for the tempo and then phrasing. I introduced six-note patterns which I reduced to four-, three- and then two-note patterns. He followed them exactly.

When I played glissandos up the piano using a sustaining pedal, he matched that by playing single beats on the cymbal.

A period of time followed, lasting about 30 seconds, when we sustained a fairly stable pattern of pulsed playing. This then generated into short phrases which he imitated and followed. He was following the melody line I was playing most effectively with his drum playing and he was also following the tempo of the melody.

I introduced a vocal idea to him, again a short phrase of three notes followed by a five-note tonal melody. He copied it, singing with me, anticipating quickly the direction of the melody. He also started to extend the melody on his own initiative, using the phrase pattern that I was singing. When I picked up his idea, he at this point voluntarily began to play the cymbal and drum again. I joined with him on the piano, again sharing the crescendo and accelerando that he was making and extending it myself, which he followed.

The final part of this first section ended with a vocal exchange where he matched very precisely the vocal ideas I was producing. We put the sticks down. I leaned across the drum towards him and he leaned towards me. I sang short four- to six-note phrases which I extended to seven- or eight-note phrases and he sang similar phrases back to me, not only matching the length of the phrases but matching the pitch. I was singing at the top of my range, so he sang in a quite high voice at the top of his range. Finally, I started drumming with my fingers on the drum, which he copied, extending it to drumming across the drum to his hands and making a game of 'animals scrambling across the drum'. As my sleeves were getting in the way, I pushed the sleeves of my jumper back up my arms, a movement which Barry immediately copied himself.

Summary of first section

The events I scored are documented on Table 4.1. The first section revealed a significant number of events I charted where Barry was following me and a lesser number where he was either partnering or taking the lead himself. In terms of variability, I found very few examples of rigid playing as Barry was so flexible and variable in the way he was playing both in terms of his tempo, the instruments he was using (timbre) and in melodic ideas. However, there was a balance of events where he maintained a stable idea and began to vary it, and a small number where he was making quite big contrasts in how he was playing.

Conclusion and interpretation of the analysis of Section 1

At this point my impression was that Barry was a child who was imitating, copying and following what I was doing for quite a large proportion of the time. However, in terms of evidence of autistic disability, there were very few examples of either rigid behaviour or resistiveness in terms of his interpersonal/interactive behaviour. On the contrary, he was following ideas well, attending quite closely to what I was doing, and already revealing a quite different level of creativity to that which had been experienced in the

Table 4.1 Improvisation Assessment Profiles

Patient's Name: ___BARRY___ *Date:* _____

ANALYSIS

Section 1: Piano+Drums; Section 2: Piano+Metallophone; Section 3: Piano duet

Autonomy   ## Variability

Dependant	1	2	3	Rigid	1	2	3
Rhythmic Ground	2	–	–	Tempo	–	–	–
Melody	3	–	–	Melody	–	–	–
Timbre	–	–	–	Timbre	–	–	–
Follower				**Stable**			
Rhythmic Ground	12	3	2	Tempo	7	3	1
Melody	6	–	–	Melody	5	2	–
Timbre	2	–	1	Timbre	2	7	–
Partner				**Variable**			
Rhythmic Ground	3	2	2	Tempo	8	5	3
Melody	1	1	3	Melody	6	3	2
Timbre	1	–	–	Timbre	8	1	5
Leader				**Contrasting**			
Rhythmic Ground	4	7	3	Tempo	3	2	2
Melody	1	4	–	Melody	1	1	3
Timbre	1	–	–	Timbre	8	1	5
Resister				**Random**			
Rhythmic Ground	–	–	4	Tempo	–	–	1
Melody	–	–	–	Melody	–	–	–
Timbre	–	–	2	Timbre	–	–	–

Source: adapted from Bruscia (1987)

speech and language therapy session and the art therapy session. Between the end of this section and the next section which I analysed was a period where I asked Barry to find the instrument under the table. Initially, I asked him without gestural or eye-pointing cues. He appeared not to understand at all what I was asking him and didn't even look at the table when I mentioned the word. He echoed what I said two or three times and it wasn't until I physically pointed to where the metallophone was under the table that he looked over. Even then he still didn't understand from my verbal suggestion that he should 'go and get the instrument under the table' that I was wanting him to do that. Based on this short exchange, it became apparent that Barry had a severe lack of understanding of language and didn't understand my question or my direction at all.

Because he had been so effective in watching me and following me during the first section, I decided at this point in the session to adopt a strategy whereby he couldn't see what I was doing, so that we would be working more independently and our level of interaction would be determined much more by sound cues than by visual cues. As long as he was watching me I had a feeling that he would follow what I was doing, either because he thought that was what he was meant to do or because it was the only way he knew how to cope with the situation. Therefore, I went over and sat at the other piano, half-turned away from him, and he was left playing the metallophone facing away from me.

Section 2

Barry started playing the metallophone and I joined in with tonal, supportive, pulsed and melodic improvised music. While initially checking over his shoulder that I was there and playing with him, Barry then didn't look round again but began to take his own initiative on how to play. Within six or seven seconds he had halved his tempo and I slowed down with him. I started to sing quietly while he was playing at this speed and he voluntarily picked up with much more confident and firm singing of his own while he was playing, singing in clear phrases. He sang a four-bar phrase, which I matched, and he also demonstrated a clear ability to form melodies inside the internal structure of a key, using a tonic as his ground and structuring his melody above and below the tonic. He spontaneously began to play with the ends of the beaters instead of the felt heads and then changed the speed to a faster tempo. He increased his volume and began to increase his tempo. He anticipated a cadence that I was making and then, after I paused, again began to spontaneously sing a melody.

What was noticeable as this improvisation progressed was that Barry was, to some extent, in his own musical world. I am sure that he could hear my support and my accompaniment because he picked up little melodic ideas from me and matched his tempo to mine after he had initiated a change. I was following him much more during this improvisation. He reached over to use the snare drum and then, hearing a short three- to four-note melodic pattern from me, began to play short patterns himself, looking over to wait until I had repeated them. This happened four times. It was also noticeable in this section that he decided when to stop and start.

At the end of this section I introduced a song that I knew he was familiar with from the television – 'Thomas the Tank Engine'. At first, he had flicked one of the keys off the metallophone, so he was a little preoccupied with replacing it and getting the one next to it correctly placed. I continued with the song on the piano and he joined in at the right tempo, playing to the end of the song. I didn't finish the tune but extemporized it into an improvisation, whereupon he began to extend onto the snare drum and introduced more of his own vocal material, singing quite loudly and clearly melodic phrases.

Scoring the number of events of both autonomy and variability, again looking at the musical elements of tempo, melody and timbre, I noted a significantly greater number of events where Barry demonstrated musical leadership (Table 4.1). There were now less events of partnership and following in this section. Barry couldn't see me and he began to organize his musical material around what he wanted to do, although there were some events where he was affected by my ideas. The variability scale revealed a balance of events between stable playing, variable and contrasting playing. There were no events that I could describe as either rigid or random in this section or in the last section, which are more typical of children who either have rather rigid and repetitive features of behaviour due to autistic disability or a chaotic way of behaving due to severe learning disability.

Section 3

The final section that I chose to analyse was a section where Barry joined me on the piano for a piano duet improvisation. Barry began by playing an ascending scale right up to the top of the piano in a steady pulse. He then developed into playing clusters of notes with a variable tempo, which I where he stopped and then played single spaced beats. A rapid succession of changes in tempo followed where he occasionally matched my tempo but frequently changed to his own speeds. He continued to play short rhythmic patterns, typically . . – or . . . – . After three minutes of playing we had a short reflective passage of slow gentle playing where I used the sustaining pedal and Barry played quite slowly and softly. He then reverted to his faster tempo, playing up and down the keys at variable speeds, using mainly two- or three-minute clusters with occasional single-note playing. What was noticeable at this point was that he had become quite independent in his playing and I was very much in the role of a follower. When he began a fixed-tempo playing, I followed and supported him with an accompaniment, but there were one or two events where he deliberately changed and moved away from the tempo I was attempting to establish. As the improvisation went on, he increasingly developed his exploration of the keyboard, particularly changing the position where he was playing on the keys. I introduced the tune 'Thomas the Tank Engine' again and he matched that with single-note playing at the same tempo in which I was playing. There were some examples in this section of resistiveness both to playing with me and one occasion when his playing became quite random on the variability profile. Towards the end he decided to work his way right down to the bottom of the keyboard, reaching across me to hit the bass keys of the piano.

In the analysis I made of the number of events in this section there were again a greater number of events where he demonstrated musical leadership and a significantly less number where he was following the ideas I was producing (Table 4.1).

Conclusion

Analysis of the data I was able to take from the three sections gave me some significant evidence of Barry's interactive abilities and his creative skills. In my report I described him in the following way:

> Barry is very interactive, makes good eye contact, tolerates physical contact and has good skills both on the instruments and in the subtleties of the communication we were sharing together. He seems to have a comprehension problem and also patterned repetitive speech at the moment. However the level of interaction was so good that I feel it definitely puts him outside the bracket of any autistic disability, and although there was some evidence of sequencing, it was not at all perseverative or obsessional, and he was easily diverted. He demonstrates

skills in turn taking, sharing, and the frequency during the improvisational music making that he was able to both follow and take the lead demonstrates his ability to operate at a partnership level. In terms of the variability of his playing, he did not demonstrate rigid or random musical playing to any significant degree, and varied between stable ideas and variable ideas.

Generally, Barry's use of the musical instruments and his way of making music with me was not congruent with musical and social behaviour one typically finds that would support a diagnosis of autism. He did not demonstrate some of the repetitive and frequently inappropriate ways of using instruments that I have come to expect from children with autistic disability. There were no examples of flicking, over-orientation on tactile experiences, spinning, sequencing or ordering, or routine bound/rigid music making. He was much more able to share the experience and anticipate and empathize with the ideas I was offering him than one would expect at a musical level in a child on the autistic spectrum.

General conclusion

Experience over the years has taught me that it is impossible to follow only a single approach, however methodologically and clinically safe that may be. Flexibility is essential in the music therapist's skills and adaptability to the clients' needs, to the situation and to their changing emotional and interactional state, within a broad but well-bounded framework, is an effective model. The approach and therapeutic intervention described above ranges from a strongly structured framework to a flexible and free style of work, and the combination of these approaches has proved effective in diagnostic assessment.

At a fundamental level, my influences have been primarily client centred and cognitive, balanced with a holistic viewpoint. With that background, I endeavour to sustain and achieve consistent support for my clients, giving them unconditional positive regard at all levels. In both assessment sessions and sustained treatment I have found the need to provide a variety of musical and interpersonal frameworks with which we can explore our relationship, the client's needs, the client's problems, and find the appropriate therapeutic direction.

Having insight into the appropriate time and place to take a more challenging approach, or when to give a strong feeling of empathy and shared feeling, is at the heart and soul of the therapist's skill and judgement. Sometimes, this is achieved by possessing and developing strong and reliable intuition, but, at the same time, intuition is influenced by previous knowledge and previous experiences and a rapid and effective process of evaluation and judgement.

The process of assessment demands both an objective and subjective attitude on the part of the music therapist. The model I have described of the structure of a therapy assessment has been developed more specifically to be used in diagnostic assessment. Therapy assessment will require more evaluation over time.

The use of the IAPs in evaluating the musical material and the interpersonal relationship gives a very musical criteria to work with in evaluating musical activity before attempting to form hypotheses, interpretations and conclusions. It is a method whereby elements in the musical material can be looked at, or focused on, in order to integrate thinking about the client's musical world. At one level I could feel inadequate, in that I have not done justice to the complexity and completeness of the IAPs and the full potential. However, this is an adaptation I have made in order to use the profiles and the scales effectively, within time constraints, to evaluate, in part, the relevant aspects of a child's musical and pathological behaviour.

There are limitations in the process I have described, and in the analysis. The primary limitation is the subjectivity with which I have undertaken the analysis and with which I have scored events. In the Harper House assessment it is possible to see the child in other assessments, therefore being better informed but also potentially biased. The process I go through to make this analysis is to review the session from memory, watch the video of the whole session in order to select the sections I want to analyse and then watch the specific sections again in order to score them, so the events I have scored are selected from, effectively, a third and fourth viewing of the session. Nevertheless, there is no inter-observer reliability and this method has not been researched to explore issues of external validity and reliability. The use I have made of this method to date is solely for clinical purposes in diagnostic assessment.

There are also limitations in the excluding and reductionist nature of the process. Music therapy improvisation provides a very rich source of material for analysis and the method I have demonstrated in using the structure I have described, followed by the analysis model using the IAPs, also relies on good judgement by the therapist to follow an appropriate and fruitful process in the session and then select relevant sections and musical elements in the scales for analysis. This also leaves one vulnerable to individual bias and selective interpretation. However, the external validation I am able to find comes in the process following the analysis and report writing. At Harper House each case will have a case co-ordinator who could be any member of the team that originally saw the child in the first appointment. Their job is to compare and contrast the findings of the various assessment reports, looking for evidence of an agreed picture of the child. The conclusions reached in the music therapy assessment using this model of analysis will be compared to other therapy assessments, and major discrepancies in interpretation or in the overall picture between disciplines can result in the need for further analysis, consideration and reconsideration. The final conclusions, written by the case co-ordinator (a role I have many times undertaken), need to reflect an agreed picture and consistent recommendations.

The techniques of the work described above represent a part of the resources that can be drawn on. It does not, by any means, cover the whole but can give some insights into the parts which make up the whole. Having said that, I would not wish anybody to regard some of the above descriptions as 'recipes' that can be easily or quickly applied in therapeutic situations. In clinical practice, and also in music therapy training, I have found that what is more significant than purely the techniques, materials and structure that goes into making up therapy is *how* you work through the process and what you yourself bring to the process. Reaching people through music is partly to do with understanding the feeling of contact from them by the music they are making, but it is also to do with joining with them in a musical experience and bringing your own music and musical personality to them.

References

Alvin, J. (1965) *Music for the Handicapped Child.* Oxford: Oxford University Press.

Alvin, J. (1975) *Music Therapy.* London: Hutchinson.

Alvin, J. (1978) *Music Therapy for the Autistic Child.* Oxford: Oxford University Press.

Beck, A.T. and Weishaar, M.E. (1989) 'Cognitive Therapy.' In R.J. Corsini and D. Wedding (eds) *Current Psychotherapies.* Illinois: Peacock Publishers Inc.

Bruscia, K. (1987) *Improvisational Models of Music Therapy.* Springfield, Illinois: Charles C. Thomas Publications.

Bruscia, K. (1991) *Case Studies in Music Therapy.* Pennsylvania: Barcelona Publishers.

Bunt, L. (1994) *Music Therapy: An Art Beyond Words.* London: Routledge.

Heal, M. and Wigram, T. (1994) *Music Therapy in Health and Education.* London: Jessica Kingsley Publishers.

John, D. (1995) 'The therapeutic relationship in music therapy as a tool in the treatment of psychosis.' In T. Wigram, B. Saperston and R. West (eds) *The Art and Science of Music Therapy: A Handbook.* London, Toronto: Harwood Academic Publications.

Nordoff, P. and Robbins, C. (1971) *Therapy in Music for Handicapped Children.* London: Victor Gollancz.

Nordoff, P. and Robbins, C. (1975) *Music Therapy in Special Education.* London: Macdonald and Evans.

Nordoff, P. and Robbins, C. (1977) *Creative Music Therapy.* New York: John Day.

Odell-Miller, H. (1995) 'Approaches to music in psychiatry with specific emphasis upon a research project with the elderly mentally ill.' In T. Wigram, B. Saperston and R. West (eds) *The Art and Science of Music Therapy: A Handbook.* London, Toronto: Harwood Academic.

Pavlicevic, M. (1995) 'Interpersonal processes in clinical improvisation; towards a subjectively systematic definition.' In T. Wigram, B. Saperston and R. West (eds) *The Art and Science of Music Therapy: A Handbook.* London, Toronto: Harwood Academic.

Pavlicevic, M. (1997) *Music Therapy in Context.* London: Jessica Kingsley Publishers.

Priestley, M. (1975) *Music Therapy in Action.* London: Constable.

Priestley, M. (1995) 'Linking sound and symbol.' In T. Wigram, B. Saperston and R. West (eds) *The Art and Science of Music Therapy: A Handbook.* London, Toronto: Harwood Academic.

Raskin, N.J. and Rogers, C. (1989) 'Person-Centered Therapy.' In R. Corsini and D. Wedding (eds) *Current Psychotherapies.* Illinois: Peacock Publishers.

Stige, B. and Ostergaard, B. (1993) *Improvisations Profiler.* Norway: Hogeskulle Saudaue.

Trevarthen, C., Aitken, K., Papoudi, D. and Robarts, J. (1996) *Children with Autism. Diagnosis and Interventions to Meet Their Needs.* London: Jessica Kingsley Publishers.

Wigram, T. (1991a) 'Music therapy for a girl with Rett's Syndrome: Balancing structure and freedom.' In K. Bruscia (ed) *Case Studies in Music Therapy.* Pennsylvania: Barcelona Publishers.

Wigram, T. (1991b) 'Die Bedeutung musikalischen Verhaltens und Empfanglichkeit im Verlauf der Differentialdiagnose von Autismus und anderen Retardierungen.' *OBM. Zietschrift Des Osterreichiscren Berufsverbands der Musiktherapeuten.* Vol. 1–91, 4–18.

Wigram, T. (1992a) 'Aspects of music therapy relating to physical disability. Keynote paper to the 1991 Annual Congress of AMTA, Sydney, Australia.' *Australian Journal of Music Therapy 3,* 3–15.

Wigram, T. (1992b) 'Differential diagnosis of autism and other types of disability. Keynote paper to the 1991 Annual Congress of AMTA, Sydney, Australia.' *Australian Journal of Music Therapy 3,* 16–26.

Wigram, T. (1995a) 'Assessment and diagnosis in music therapy.' In T. Wigram, B. Saperston and R. West (eds) *The Art and Science of Music Therapy: A Handbook.* London, Toronto: Harwood Academic Publications.

Wigram, T. (1997) 'Musicoterapia: Estructura y flexibilidad en el proceso de musicoterapia.' In P. del Campo (ed) *La Musica como Proceso Humano.* Salamanca: Amaru Ediciones.

Wigram, T., Saperston, B. and West, R. (eds) (1995) *The Art and Science of Music Therapy: A Handbook.* London, Toronto: Harwood Academic Publications.

CHAPTER 5

Music and Autism

Vocal Improvisation as Containment of Stereotypies

Gianluigi di Franco

Introduction

This chapter is focused upon music and autism considered as two codes and two languages, both able to establish a relationship between the internal world of a human being and the external environment in a considerably different way.

It is obvious that any relationship between two individuals (i.e., A and B) implies positive and/or negative aspects. Therefore, it is possible that a positive connection between A and B can be set up, but it is also possible that A withdraws and expresses negatively and unconsciously his unavailability to a contact with inward and outward realities. Consequently, he works out a kind of special and incomprehensible code for B. This attitude may be considered a 'bizarre' expression of his own self and not necessarily an attempt of establishing a bilateral communication. However, the following remarks might fit both codes:

A. Music is an expressive language made of sounds which can have different degrees of emotional significance on cognitive and emotional levels.

B. Autism is an unconscious way to express, through a 'bizarre' attitude, the capability the exploded SELF has not only to be a NOT-SELF, but, in any case, a SELF.

Moreover, music and autism share common regressive aspects. Music has the potential to help human beings in reaching deep regressional stages and autism is a sort of prototypical regressive condition determined by biologic and/or psychological reasons.

It must be added that autism has been described also as a moment in the development of human beings according to the three stages described by Mahler (1972): a first stage defined as normal autism (until six years old); a second stage defined as normal symbiosis (from six years old to twelve) and a third stage defined as separation – individuation (from twelve years old to eighteen).

Such remarks are the result of a period of observation lasting eight years and carried out with clients diagnosed as having primary autism or secondary autism (i.e., produced by another pathology, often a neurologic disorder).

It is clear that it would be a mistake to classify music and autism in the same way, even though it is possible to find common features in the dynamics of both.

If we consider the DSM-IV for developmental generalized disturbances and, particularly, the F.84.0 Autistic Disturbance (299.00), it is then possible to elicit what follows:

A. 1 d) lack of emotional reciprocity;

    2 a) lack of or delay in spoken language

    2 a) stereotyped and repetitive or bizarre language

    3 c) stereotyped motor rituals

B. 3) delay or lack of physiological functioning within a capability of symbolic or imaginative play. However, two other important components must be considered together with the above mentioned ones, that is:

    a) lack of emotional significances

    b) more or less structured stereotyped activities as significant memories.

It is necessary to point out that motor stereotyped activities and repetitive activities, which are central for the symptomatology of autism, do not have to be considered as equal, especially taking into account the peculiarities of both. The following definitions will help the understanding of these differences:

Repetitiveness: the client's tendency to present a behavioural attitude originating in a compulsive need

Rigidity: the client's tendency to carry out a behaviour always in the same way, which comes from a poor flexibility in motor actions as well as in thinking.

Persistency: the client's tendency to perpetuate a behaviour, caused by his difficulty in breaking with routine.

Repetitiveness is the feature which is much closer to the clinical aspects of autism. The compulsive need originates in an attitude of extreme defence against being in contact with two important and dynamic aspects inherent in a more balanced way of communicating. They imply that repeating an action means to move away from the emotional significance which could be pertinent to that specific moment and repeating the same action several times creates also a barrier between one's own self and another self.

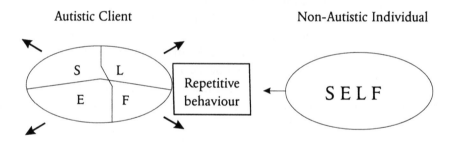

Figure 5.1 Repetitiveness (defence of exploded self)

The autistic client repeats actions. In so doing he expresses an exploded Self that works out iterative patterns in motor and thinking structures within a fusional habitat in order to be more defended from the possibility of developing an awareness of his own self (HIM-SELF) than from establishing relationships with another self, or, as Donna Williams (1998) states, with a 'SELF-STATE' or 'SELF-NESS'.

However, this relationship is inevitably based on his bizarre way of functioning, moving, speaking and not being involved on an emotional level. Therefore, it could be said that the peculiarities of the autistic behaviour for active productions are mirrored by stereotyped patterns. On the other hand, stereotyped movements and thoughts are tightly connected with the main elements in music and, particularly, with rhythm.

It would be useful at this point to take into account the contributions given by various disciplines to this same subject:

> *Anthropology:* '…stereotyped activities can be the signs of a confinement due to suffering…' (Barlow 1977, p.47)

> *Psychoanalysis:* '…an obsession, an action, a sequence of behaviours can be defined as being compulsive when a failure in their fulfilment is felt as a reason for reinforcing them…the client does not remember anything about what he forgot…but he acts it out. He reproduces sequences not as memories but as actions. He repeats them without knowing that he is repeating them…' (Freud 1914, p.150)

> *Psychology:* '…the act of repeating implies a feeling of gratification due to expectations or a feeling of wonder for unexpected events, both caused by renewing the same things over and over or by variations in them…' (Fraisse 1974, p.176). And always in Fraisse's book, titled *Psychology of the Rhythm*' it is stressed that 'the concept of rhythm would not be originated by experiences in nature but by the organization of human movement'. Also, Nach (1865) considers motor activities as central for our experiences in rhythm. And, again quoting from Fraisse (1974): 'Consequently he looks for the origin of subjective accentuation which is perceived when one listens attentively to a sequence of sounds objectively equal as for the motor actions accompanying them…' (p.176)

Moreover, it is possible to add other remarks in order to underline the close connection between repeated motor actions and rhythm. For instance, Burns (1930) states that 'rhythm is the expression of order and symmetry' (see pp. 63–66); Peiper (1937) maintains that 'there is a connection between the nervous centre which controls the movements of children's sucking and the centre of breath and because of such connection the movements of sucking soon become rhythmical according to breath' (see pp.201–206) and Yates (1935) states that 'the rhythmical patterns acquired during the first months of life have to be considered as the basis for the perception of time and rhythm' (see pp.341–355).

The ideas expressed in these quotations, which have been taken from the works of authors with different backgrounds, help our understanding of autistic clients. For instance, the reason why the autistic client performs repetitive actions is explained. It lies in his effort of balancing defensively his confinement, a place where he stays trying to keep himself as far as possible from pain. Then the method he uses to handle his ability to express himself is to reproduce materials not as memories, thus involving his affectivity, but as actions, thus going back to the primary levels of developmental processes, as Piaget described, at a time when the mental process of symbolization was not yet structured. The process of symbolization implies having memories and all the emotional aspects related to them. Therefore, if an individual has problems with the emotional significance of a certain symbol, he can go back and establish a contact, not a relationship, with that object as an object and not as a thing from which a memory could be evoked thanks to perceptions and emotions. Moreover, when working with an autistic client it could be useful to start trying to get into his 'closed circle' and, in so doing, to create, through a primitive and almost unstructured musical framework, a feeling of gratification for the expectation of something and a feeling of wonder for unexpected events.

I would like to discuss some relevant points of the approach I use in my work in music therapy before presenting some clinical cases, mainly focused on stereotypies, as prominent symptomatologic aspects of clients diagnosed as autistic.

Philosophy and theoretical orientation for clinical practice

The use of sounds is mainly aimed at fostering the individual's 'overall' ability of expression in communication.

The language of sounds combines all the possibilities of using, living and interacting with sounds, which frees them from the limitations of a formal and aesthetic ideal and/or an analytical and structural conception and gives value to concrete sounds, sounds of nature, biological sounds, folkloric sounds and instrumental sounds.

Therefore, music therapy is a discipline which uses sound musical language in a dual or group relationship as a means (not as an aim) within a systematic process of intervention with preventive, rehabilitative and therapeutic goals. Music therapy is often provided together with other therapies in order to achieve common goals.

All the pathologies treated with music therapy are connected with communication both for the cognitive and the affective areas.

Music therapy uses several techniques, according to the different issues in the area of expression concerning a certain pathology. However, all of them aim at releasing, melting and amplifying expressive and communication blocks.

First of all, my approach in music therapy is mainly holistic. The general aim is to establish a wide and containing relationship with the client as a human being and then to focus on the specific symptoms, working through sounds. Second, all this occurs within a context which is observed from inside and outside for its implications (musical as well as relational implications). It is an evolutive context in which the development of the musical activity is updated and tuned with the events which occur within what I define as a 'music therapy relationship'.

Methodology of intervention

The three basic stages foreseen in my clinical practice are as follows:

(1) SOUND ANAMNESIS (Assessment)

    1a. *Interview* with the client's family, with or without the client. It consists of collecting data during an interview concerning:

- the clinical diagnosis
- parallel activities carried out by the client
- musical-sound profile of the client's family
- musical-sound profile of the client.

    1b. *A receptive test* to assess the client's cognitive and emotional reactions to pre-recorded sound fragments (three minutes each with intervals between each fragment of about three minutes):

- a rhythmic fragment (binary)
- a melodic fragment (aleatory – instrumental fragments are preferred)
- a harmonic fragment (polyphonic with voice)
- an electronic fragment (electronic sounds with different dynamics and intensity)
- sounds from nature.

Instruments representing the different instrumental categories are available to the client.

The therapist here acts as an observer and does not participate.

1c. *Three active tests:*

- a rhythmical test (binary and ternary cells)
- a melodic test (third, fifth and seventh intervals)
- a harmonic test (popular harmonic tunes in major and minor modes).

These tests assess the client's reactions to active production. The therapist plays a 'directive' role with his proposals to the client, assessing the extent to which the client reacts to a relationship (transference) with the therapist, the objects and the working milieu. These tests are interpreted according to the following parameters:

- level of sound production and listening
- favourite instruments
- ability of responding to stimuli
- intensity – tone/pitch – timbre
- psychomotor ability
- ways of relating to objects
- ability of potential communication
- ways of interacting with others
- production of rhythmic cells
- production of melodic fragments
- production of harmonic sequences.

It is possible at this stage to assess both the quantitative aspects (musical-sound implications) and the qualitative aspects (relational implications) and to create a working hypothesis using the collected data. Such a hypothesis takes into account:

- an area of intervention
- period of the intervention
- different phases

- goals
- kind of setting.

A working methodology which takes into account:

- the musical techniques which have been used
- the roles played by the therapist.

Such a working methodology is based on a psychodynamic approach and refers particularly to psychoanalysis which provides the guidelines for:

(2) a phase of OBSERVATION.

(3) a phase of CLINICAL EVALUATION.

The phase of observation follows the lines of a basic protocol to which specific points for each treated pathology are added. The evaluation in each session includes the following points:

- the position of the body with regard to the instruments
- the choice of the instruments and the meaning of such a choice
- mimical and gestural aspects
- musical dynamics as for intensity – tone/pitch – timbre
- emotional ways of approaching the instruments
- ways of performing with the instruments (traditional or non-traditional ways of handling the instruments)
- description of rhythmic cells
- description of melodic phrases
- description of harmonic sequences
- interaction between rhythm, melody and harmony
- the sound ability of integrating with another individual or of denying another individual
- the ability of living silence as a musical pause
- attention abilities to the sound stimuli
- the ability of listening to oneself and to others
- sound dialogue (ways of dialogue pertinent to rhythmical cells, melodic phrases and/or harmonic sequences) – imitation,

alternation (turn taking, questions and answers), overlap (overlapping of questions and answers)

- parallel creative aspects (painting, dance, verbalization, etc.)
- the ability of slowing down or speeding up a melodic phrase and/or a rhythmic cell
- individuation of the favourite object-instrument for expressing and communicating (intermediary object/transitional object)
- description of the therapist's countertransference
- diagram of the movements in space which occurred in each session to the most meaningful moments in sound communication.

The development of the process takes into account the 'here-and-now' moments of significance of each session, within which the sound space is used in order to engage and develop relationships.

Moreover, each 'here-and-now' moment is observed from the outside as for the occurred events (second position). Such events are considered in connection with the established goals and the techniques. A supervisor (third position, as neutral one) is often provided to contain and solve the issues concerning the therapist's professional ability (therapist-centred supervision) or to contain and solve the issues concerning a client who is undergoing a treatment procedure (client-centred supervision).

All the various 'here-and-now' events are then evaluated according to a longitudinal perspective in which each moment is perceived as a development and growth and in which each moment is already contained in the one which follows (as in Chinese boxes). This process aims at evaluating and testing the effectiveness of the treatment with regard to the established goals.

The dynamic process within the relationship foresees an *imitation phase* followed by a *dialogic phase* and, particularly, a sound holding phase in which the therapist tries to develop an awareness of the sound material brought by the client, 'supports' him physically and, therefore, holds him; an imitation and assimilation phase in which the therapist considers the sound production of the 'here-and-now' moments going back to the sound memory of a developing relationship and enriching the already existing sound relationship – this is the case when the therapist performs a 'maternage' function through sounds and a dialogic relationship phase in which the therapeutic relationship develops from a primitive 'fusional phase' to a relationship where creative actions are fostered in order to facilitate individuation processes. Here the therapist uses 'themes' to improvise and create sound dialogues.

Music therapy work with pathologies connected with communication at the deepest level can result in regressive reactions linked to the sound-lived experiences. They can be contained partly by the work of the therapist in the 'here-and-now' situations and partly by diacritic supervision, in which the supervisor's role is to intervene from the outside in a neutral way on the work of the therapist.

The music therapy relationship refers to the setting as a communication system in which there are opposite possibilities to be tested, such as: a linear bi-uniform communication in which a verbal or sound message produced by A can easily be understood and decoded by B and, therefore, B can answer to A, making him realize that he understood his message; a star-like communication in which the features and the elements of A's language are open towards different directions and, therefore, cannot be easily understood by B, who can be reached only by a split part of A's expressive production.

It is advisable for a therapist who develops an awareness of a star-like communication to start from a similar position in order to catch at least a communicative fragment, to make it acquire a meaning through a transitional area in which sound games become central.

The role of the music therapist is connected to the different pathologies and to them being more or less severe as indicated by the assessment. It tends to be 'semi-directive' and the therapist generally follows the following guidelines:

- mainly listens during the first stages
- acts as a selecting filter for listening, according to the data collected from the sound anamnesis and the first meetings, with a view to catching a communication fragment conveyed by the client
- proposition/imitative response
- proposition/improvised response
- proposition/dialogue.

Vocal techniques

I would like to provide some fundamental elements of the musical techniques which can help working on motor stereotypies and/or stereotyped attitude, both connected with autism.

A topical use of voice and vocalization together with instruments which represent all the categories of instruments, is looked at as a technical approach (Di Franco 1995). Such a method has to be tested and evaluated for its pertinence within a given process.

The use of voice is advisable since it is connected with the use of the body as an object-instrument and, therefore, facilitates bodily contact so that it is possible to intervene directly on motor stereotypies.

The use of voice opens a channel for rhythmic and melodic patterns which facilitate sound communication in situations where the therapist's body is 'engaged' in a fusional and symbiotic relation and, therefore, other possibilities cannot be explored.

The use of voice helps moving from one moment to another in the session. The vocal expression is, therefore, a 'bridge' and a support for other sound events.

This modality proposes what can follow: imitating the instrumental and/or vocal fragment produced by the client as for its intensity, pitch, timbre and rhythm; producing variations of this same fragment, such as dividing the musical phrase rhythmically, making melodic variations, making harmonies proceeding in thirds, fifths, sevenths and octaves, and going back to the original tonality.

The above-mentioned aspects have been related to the intensity (pp/p/mp/f/ff), the rhythmic pace (speeding up/slowing down) and to different kinds of interactive frameworks.

The vocal improvisation takes different shapes, such as lullabies, rough songs, structured songs and songs with lyrics.

Clinical cases

I would like to present here two short vignettes and a longer case study of autistic clients with whom I have worked clinically. My point is to show and discuss differences in these autistic 'worlds' according to the ways these clients have to express themselves, the musical modalities used to approach them, the dynamic processes within the relationships, different diagnosis of different autistic states and common and different ways used by the clients to express themselves through repetitive patterns.

The first case of autism regards Antonio (14 years old), diagnosed as having primary autism since he was three years old. He began a music therapy treatment two-and-a-half years ago and was referred by a psychologist who had observed that he had a nice musical sensitivity. First, I had to find out if there were common points or areas of lack of understanding. He was very fluent in musical production and I was impressed by his way of performing and because I did not get the impression of him being so autistic within music. Then I started to analyse my counter-transference and had to adopt the behavioural attitude of a professional musician, since he was so capable in music, in order to develop an awareness of his problems (and, in some respects, also, of my own problems). He was trying all the time to show the extent to which he was able to perform traditional and well-known songs, even though it was much more aimed at strengthening his identity than at confirming his narcissistic drives. Playing together during this first stage, where I performed the role of the musician, was very effective. He felt that the competition was hard to win but he had found a friend.

The second clinical case regards Giuseppe (9 years old), diagnosed as having primary autism. He began a treatment in music therapy three years ago. His referral to music therapy was due to a need for containing him since he was hyperactive and aggressive to others. During a first working stage he showed the following characteristics: echolalia, dissociative thinking, a high level of hyperactivity and stereotyped patterns. Therefore, he was offered just a few instruments and a type of semi-directive approach was chosen in order to give him a chance of expressing himself, but, at the same time, to become aware of the existence of boundaries in the space where he was acting, in the time in which he was acting and for the objects he was developing an awareness of.

As I mentioned before, my work was mostly oriented to containing this client and not to getting inside a such repetitive and unstructured circle. As the intensity of his stereotyped activity lowered, I started to reflect some of the patterns he reproduced, trying to make little changes which were not melodic or rhythmical but were concerned with the intensity of the sounds, the use of different instruments and playing back to him the codes he had brought into the session. He was caught by this modality and, from that moment on, he became more balanced in his way of performing and paid more attention to what I was doing, so creating more pauses for silence. He had broken his hyperactivity pattern, giving his silence the value of a musical pause.

The third clinical case regards Fabio (9 years old), diagnosed as having primary autism. He began music therapy treatment when he was six years old. At the moment he has given it up because of family problems. This is the most severe case among the ones discussed here since it involves a case of classical autism as described in DSM-IV. Fabio was referred by a clinician in a town located in central Italy, who suggested music therapy as the *'extrema ratio'*.

SOUND ANAMNESIS (first contact with the client)

21/02/1995
Name: Fabio
Sex: Male
Age: 6
Diagnosis of referral: Autistic psychosis
Results of the musical tests

1   Reaction to the sound fragments

> He shows interest in the shape and the sound of almost all the proposed instruments.

2   Production/Listening

> F. tends to make isolated and microscopic productions; He is available to listening activities but only when he is guided or he is curious at a particular sound and of the movement connected to its production.

3   Favourite instruments

> F. prefers instruments with acute frequencies and loud and very loud volume; the instruments he chooses are crotala, triangles and cymbals.

4   Ability of becoming active

> F. is available to dynamic activities but just for a few seconds. Therefore, he sets up activities to stop immediately after.

5   Level of sound production

>   F. prefers to work with the following volumes: forte, fortissimo, mezzo forte. This is what shakes him, but this is also what shakes, above all, the other people; this obviously activates him expressively.

6   Psychomotor abilities level

>   Very good. F. shows an ability to make movements in which there is a control on posture and a good balance in walking. It is necessary to stress that when he discovers that he can go out of the boundaries, and this is due to expressive and communicational needs, he tends to throw himself down to the floor in order to be supported. He also shows a tendency to overcome the limits indicated in his working space, for instance going in and out of the music therapy room, so trying to interrupt the therapy.

7   Ways of relating to objects

>   F. starts looking for the objects but perhaps showing his fear of breaking them (during the first session he cried because he made the metallophone fall to the ground, perhaps expressing his feeling of being guilty without any possibility of repairing what he had done). He tends to manipulate the objects in order to acquire an awareness of them. He manipulates them in a traditional way from a musical point of view even though, often, they become part of symbolic games.

8   Ability of potential communication

>   F. has a wide range of expression which is not specifically related to sound production but is very much based on the 'challenge' connected to the relationship he establishes.

9   Ways of interacting with other people

>   He showed a partial emotional investment towards the therapist even though this has to be investigated more.

His mother has been present in all the assessment sessions apart from the last one. This was required by the therapist because he wanted to check if Fabio's going in and out of the therapy room was connected with his mother's presence. The result was that Fabio stayed in the therapy room for longer when his mother is not there.

Work perspectives

Quantitative aspects (sound – musical productions) and Qualitative aspects (interactive implications):

- F. is a child who is sensitive to the production of sounds, therefore it is possible to work with him with music therapy.

- He is interested in the instruments which produce loud volume and he does not reject the use of the voice. His being available has to be evaluated on a quantitative level regarding expression since he produces only for a few moments without staying on the specific aspects that he himself begins.

- F. offers the possibility of working physically, therefore it is possible to formulate a hypothesis of approach with movement and rhythm.

- F. shows his major difficulties for the boundaries time and space. He does not see the therapy room as a working space and therefore tends to go in and out of the setting, and he does not give the feeling of referring to a time process but functions according to an expressive 'brainstorming'.

- During the receptive test F. showed a listening ability which made him feel emotionally moved particularly during the listening activity of the melodic and harmonic fragments.

Working hypothesis and methodology

This is the central point of the music therapy work since F. refers to very strong bipolar behaviour which make his 'containment' difficult in spite of his potential availability and the impression he gives to be able to invest his affection in the therapist.

A first period of treatment of four months, twice a week is suggested for this client in order to check how he can use the experience in music therapy and considering the above-mentioned characteristics (on suggestion of the neuropsychiatrist C. Vittozzi who referred him to music therapy).

A setting structured in two ways from the musical point of view is suggested for Fabio:

1   improvisation

2   listening.

It is necessary to use melodic pieces of music in order to engage him and to improvise working with his pertinent behaviours. The aim is to provide a structure to the expressive little productions conveyed by F. and arrange them into a wider frame of communicative possibilities. The perspective is to give him boundaries which are defined by the structure of the setting and the position of the therapist in a way that he can be led back to a precise time and space within which he can have the possibility of:

- being more fluid in his expression in communicating and therefore being more oriented

- feeding and widening production and listening channels through a musical-sound language starting from the basic level offered by F. during the assessment.

I started treatment with Fabio with a listening activity of a selection of different pieces of music which had been picked up after a sound anamnesis. Such assessment revealed that Fabio was moved only when he listened to the songs of an Italian pop singer, Amedeo Minghi, who is the author of 'easy listening' pieces of music and who uses the melodic structure of operas, namely Puccini's operas. When I started the listening activity, I presented several songs, among which there were excerpts from Puccini's operas. This activity helped him in making the decision to come to music therapy sessions, even though, for a long time (6 months), he laid on a mat in a fusional attitude with his thumb in his mouth, seldom moving, with some cold tears running on his little face. He showed no interest for the instruments as objects but he was interested in other things in the room, like papers or the clothes I was wearing. When I tried a listening activity based on pre-recorded rhythmic songs, he became more anxious and motor stereotypies appeared. I was worried about what his reactions could mean. My goal was to change his motor and ritualistic productions into more oriented activities, into a sort of musical production closer to a more balanced and understandable way of communicating, in which the object of music, like a transitional object within a developmental and warm relationship, could determine a closeness between the musical sound patterns and some possible emotional significance.

During this second working phase Fabio began to leave his structured motor stereotyped activities and to replace them with stereotyped attitudes. Therefore, he started experimenting with the objects, observing them, touching them and playing with them. At first, he was attracted by a little melodic instrument with holes like a flute, then by the keyboard. He became more uninhibited and used to play the keyboard with his feet, almost showing that he knew that his way of playing would make me 'suffer', but it was also his feeling of having a personal identity. During the following working phase he used the keyboard in a more traditional way, playing with his hands, experimenting with different sounds, sustaining notes and chords. He kept on showing his stereotyped attitudes within these more and more structured activities, repeating, for example, the same pattern many times.

At this moment he has gained more balance in his expression, he has less motor stereotyped activities and he does not have postural regressions on the floor any more.

Observation and evaluation protocols concerning this third clinical case are reported below.

Fabio has received music therapy treatment since March 1995 (see sound anamnesis) for an initial period of three months, once-a-week for 40 minutes, then twice-a-week for 25 minutes and, lately, 30 minutes for each session.

The client has been referred to music therapy by C. Vittozzi for a period of three months in order to test if such an intervention could fit in the overall treatment of this client. Music therapy treatment was approved to continue after the first three months following the report given to the referral doctor about the results of this first period of treatment.

Fabio is a client who needed to develop an awareness of the environment for a long period of time (about 3 months) in order to be able to refer to objects and situations with which he could interact and through which he could show 'fragmented elements of expression to communicate'.

Fabio becomes almost automatically attentive when listening to melodic pieces of music, during which he often tends to have regressive attitudes (he lies in a foetal position with his thumb in his mouth).

Fabio's active attention is conditioned by the 'directive' intervention of the therapist, who calls him back to a more specific involvement using sound production which is not connected to his 'ISO' (the same or similar) characteristics (Benezon 1983) and respects the rhythmical and melodic cells produced within the music therapy relationship until that moment (sound memory).

Observation parameters

POSITION OF THE CLIENT'S BODY WITH REGARD TO THE INSTRUMENTS AND THE SURROUNDING SPACE

Fabio does not use the objects in an appropriate way, but within the music therapy setting he learned:

- to turn the tape recorder on to ask for 'music'
- to accept the limits of the setting (duration 30 minutes), to stay in the space referring or not referring to the objects/instruments offered
- to refer to the music therapist as the object of the sound relationship.

Fabio tends to take postural positions which result in his body and his expressions becoming definitely 'closed', and to adopt sensitive attitudes towards sound and motor stimulation proposed by the therapist, where it is possible to see that the time he is able to sustain listening and activity has increased (from isolated moments up to 2 or 3 minutes).

Fabio tends to treat the objects/instruments as elements on which he transfers a need for containing and managing his anxiety, including them into ritual formulas such as dragging them along the floor or in the air.

THE CHOICE OF INSTRUMENT

Fabio has used melody since the beginning. Therefore, he is much more attracted to working with the voice and some simple harmonic instruments, such as the kalimba and the Russian harp, and to conveying rhythmical accents through his body.

THE MIMIC ASPECTS, GESTURES

Fabio still presents several motor stereotypies. He raises his right hand close to his right eye and laterally; he drags along oblique objects on the floor and in the air; he moves along a horizontal line with a 'rocking' movement.

When he is called back to being active, in spite of the fact that he must come to terms in order to 'adhere' to a weak relationship, he succeeds in experiencing moments in which he directs his gaze towards the therapist; greets when he arrives and when he goes away by beating the therapist's hand with his hand; and spontaneously searches for the therapist's body as a means for his need of motor expression.

THE MUSICAL DYNAMICS (INTENSITY/TONAL PITCH/TIMBRE, ETC.)

Intensity

There has been an increasing progression from this point of view. At the beginning Fabio spontaneously turns the tape recorder on to start the music, taking a position of 'withdrawn listening', after which he becomes more sensitive to the sound stimuli proposed by the therapist. Therefore, from an intensity '0' connected to the listening activity, we go towards a Medium (M) and Loud (L) intensity without reaching a Very Loud intensity.

Pitch

When Fabio started using his voice, after a period of about two-and-a-half months, we realized that he was able to sing in tune. In other words, while he was producing melodic fragments, both imitating the therapist or spontaneously referring to the implications of a sound memory developed within the music therapy relationship, he showed that he had a good level of perception of what is defined in music as tonal pitch. The discovery of this aspect provides potential for him to go further into its development.

Timbre

Fabio uses his voice in the same way a boy of his age would do, but, when he is engaged, he also experiments with different frequencies and a deeper timbre. He enjoys reproducing octaves and passes from the treble octave typical of his age to the lower one which goes towards a more adult male voice.

WAYS OF APPROACHING THE INSTRUMENT

Fabio produces spontaneously only with his voice. He seems to be suspicious of the other instruments but he uses a Russian harp, a kalimba, whistles and, sometimes, a flute and contralto tone bars. He uses other instruments, such as a tambourine or a tambourine with bells and mallets, only when there is a 'direction' on the part of the therapist. At the beginning he used the mallets to put them in his mouth, so stimulating his oral feelings. This behaviour disappeared after about two months.

WAYS OF PERFORMING WITH THE INSTRUMENTS

Fabio shows he knows how to hold an object, even though this is aimed at a simple contact with the object itself and not at being able to use it. He is never aggressive in this respect. He tries to use oblong objects in a ritualistic way. This has come to be an anchor for him to hold on to and is easily detectable from his expressive scheme.

DEVELOPMENT OF RHYTHMIC AND MELODIC INTERACTION

Fabio is not able to connect these two levels. He succeeds in producing a rhythmic cell when the therapist asks him to do so but his cell is not matching rhythmically the proposed rhythm. He succeeds in producing isolated and fragmented vocal sounds (punctiform vocal sounds) until he develops small melodic sequences which are tuned, but not connected, to a definite rhythm. He is able to detect the tone when the therapist reminds him of a precise melodic phrase.

SOUND ABILITY OF INTEGRATING WITH OTHER PEOPLE, SHARING OR DENYING THE OTHER THROUGH SOUNDS

Fabio's integration is referred to very primitive moments of fusional bodily contact and a more definite frontal exchange (when required by the therapist) in which he is much more oriented to accept such a level.

As for the sounds, Fabio still uses *imitation*, which is a point of reference for him even though there are also isolated moments of clearness in his attitude towards the other and direction in his actions. In these moments the sound language becomes an important aspect of stability.

His basic tendency is not to respond to the other, even though there are sequences he uses which give the impression of going towards the other, moving on a neutral background where his self is not characterized.

ABILITY TO SUSTAIN SILENCE

Fabio is able to sustain silence, which was the only existing element at the beginning of the therapy. Today, silence is experienced as the result of a moment of regression, a way to accompany his motor movements, which is another moment of the sound-lived experience. Silence is never, or almost never, experienced as a pause/silence within a structured musical production.

ABILITY TO BE ATTENTIVE TO SOUNDS

Fabio never, or almost never, gives the impression of paying attention to sounds but it is clear that he receives and perceives them since he often produces melodic cells which have been worked out in the previous weeks. It is as if his ability of paying attention is there but his way of expression follows different paths which do not cope directly with the events that cause them and the person with whom he can interact.

ABILITY TO LISTEN TO HIMSELF AND TO OTHER PEOPLE

Fabio listens to the pieces of music that he himself starts on the tape recorder. He is not able to listen to himself normally but, maybe, he is starting to do it through the therapist.

ABILITY TO BE ACTIVE IN TURN TAKING, TO WAIT FOR ONE'S OWN TURN AND TO RESPECT IT

Fabio does not have such abilities since he is still in a phase in which he draws things out of himself more than spending energy as regards the other.

ABILITY TO ELABORATE IN A PARALLEL WAY TO MUSICAL-SOUND ACTIVITIES

Fabio presents as an 'accurate' child in this respect. He is not invasive. He does not break the objects, but, if this happens, he feels regretful. He is not active on any level except the already described motor and sound level.

WIDENING OF THE SOUND SPACE AND ITS POSSIBLE NARROWING

Fabio is able to detect some sound cells but he does not show any remarkable ability for developing variations on the theme and/or improvisations on the same theme.

INTERMEDIARY OBJECT

Voice is Fabio's intermediary object at the moment. This is the object on which he is able to invest his affection, which also gives him the possibility to have an easier relationship with other people.

Conclusions

The interest here, from the point of view of the application of musical methodologies, lies in the feeling of gratification for the expectation that something is expressed through the voice while the movements are combined with renewing the same rhythmic/melodic cells and the possible implication of musical changes.

The compulsive behaviour is worked through by avoiding the instruments and focusing on the body and its expression through the voice. The more Fabio succeeds in making this work central, the more the rigidity of musical patterns diminishes and opens to musical variations.

It would be useful at this point to stress again some technical points which can be elicited from the above-mentioned four clinical cases of autism. The therapist who works with autistic clients should:

- tolerate silence
- tolerate unproductive situations
- tolerate repetitive activities
- tolerate more or less overall unemotional involvement
- tolerate bizarre ways of expression
- tolerate echolalias.

The therapist should establish a relationship with autistic clients mainly through:

- simple rhythmic/melodic cells
- concrete sounds (sounds produced by objects, biological sounds, sounds of nature)
- fluid sounds (water)
- sounds produced by objects which can be easily manipulated.

The therapist should use:

- a semi-directive approach
- an open approach.

He should not use a strictly directive approach which would result in making the stereotyped autistic attitudes more rigid, so running the risk of achieving the opposite goal.

The therapist should use the following musical techniques:

- listening (first stage – holding)
- mirroring (second stage – imitation)
- improvisation (third stage – dialogue).

The therapist should know the areas pertinent to autism which can be treated with music therapy, that is:

- emotional reciprocity
- eye contact
- other mimical and postural aspects (reducing movements of rocking and waving)
- partial or overall disappearance of stereotyped rituals
- increase of emotional significance within the relationship
- a better level of socialization
- possible improvement of spoken language
- possible reduction of echolalia
- a better awareness of the symbolic play.

The evaluation criteria used in the measurement of the clinical evolution of autistic pathologies should focus on stereotyped activities, with particular attention given to:

- *Features of stereotyped activities:*
  - as regards the client's body
  - as regards the other's body
  - as regards peculiar objects
  - others.
- *Emotional conditions in the course of stereotyped activities:*
  - passivity
  - well-being
  - tension

- ◦ excitement
- ◦ curiosity
- ◦ anxiety
- ◦ anguish.
- *Involvement:*
  - ◦ strong
  - ◦ moderate
  - ◦ weak.
- *Frequence:*
  - ◦ low
  - ◦ moderate
  - ◦ high.
- *Duration:*
  - ◦ low
  - ◦ moderate
  - ◦ high.

Glossary

Bi-uniform linear communication: a message conveyed by a subject A is understandable by a subject B, who can answer and receive an answer in return. Communication means can be various, such as sign language or musical-sound language.

Containment: the warm feeling of protection originating in a subject when working through a musical-sound language and its potential for regression, which leads this same subject to have himself held within.

Holding phase: the phase in which the sounds are organized with a view to contain the direct or indirect request of the subject to be in the physical and symbolic space of the relationship.

Maternage function: containing function performed through sound cells related to those primitive and fusional needs which make the therapist play a mother role – that is, to feed/breastfeed, holding the subject within its body-object. Such a function does not have to involve the therapist physically but, especially in cases in which the client is a child, it is difficult to distinguish the real form from the symbolic level and, therefore, there will be a need for giving a physical containment which can mediate the abilities for abstraction and elaboration towards the undertaking of a symbolic level.

Music therapy relationship: from a quantitative perspective, the relationship between the client and the therapist as sounds emerge within the working space and, from a qualitative perspective, the dynamics related to the exchange between the two people implied in the relationship itself.

Regression: defence mechanism existing within the contact with sounds as an unavoidable implication of deep emotional levels 'controlled' by the normal or 'pathological' resistances developed by an individual.

Significant/significance: the use of these two terms in music therapy is borrowed from F. De Saussure's (1991) use of these two concepts in linguistics. Here, in musical language, the significant could refer to the symbolic/affective value behind that same significance. These two concepts are of crucial importance for a methodological orientation in music therapy focused on the relationship level, where the connection between significants and significances in musical language can be more or less strong or, sometimes, even non-existent.

Star-like communication: the language used by a subject A within a conventional system which leads him to express himself through bizarre ways that are not understandable by a subject B (the therapist). This therapist will have to adopt a similar way of expression in order to engage even one of the fragments conveyed by A and, possibly, to communicate through it. Star-like communication means that the message conveyed by A does not follow open courses but follows different directions which are not necessarily connected, and, therefore, are not understandable by B, who does not receive integrated elements of communication but disintegrated ones.

Systematic intervention process: refers to the idea that the use of sound musical-sound language in the relationship is not a value examining one single event. But the longitudinal perspective of the different events place the one within the other, as in Chinese boxes, within a systematic process related to the communication problem in evaluation and the obtained results.

References

Barlow, G.W. (1977) 'Modal action patterns in T.A.' In Sebock (ed) *How Animals Communicate.* Bloomington: Indiana University Press.

Benenzon, R.O. (1983) *Manuale di Musicoterapia.* Rome: Borla.

Burns, C. (1930) *Movement and Types in Children.* London: Psyche.

De Saussure, F. (1993) *Corso di Linguistica Generale.* Rome: Laterza.

Di Franco, G. (1995) 'Il grido universale: Cre-azione verso una metodologia in Musicoterapia in Italia' In G. Di Franco and R. De Michele (eds), *Atti del Primo Congresso Nazionale CONFIAM.* Naples: Idelson.

Fraisse, P. (1974) *Psicologia del Ritmo.* Rome: Armando.

Freud, S. (1914) *Ricordare, Ripetere, Rielaborare.* Turin: Boringhieri.

Mahler, M. (1972) *Simbiosis Humana: les Vicisitudes de la Individuacion. Psicosis infantil.* Mexico: J. Mortiz.

Peiper, A. (1937) *Die Erseiheimung der Dominant und die Erregungsstufen des Saugzentrums.* Kinderhellk.

Williams, D. (1998) *Autism: An Inside-Out Approach.* London: Jessica Kingsley Publishers.

Yates, S. (1935) 'Some aspects of time difficulties and their relation to music.' *Journal of Psychoanalysis.*

CHAPTER 6

Islanders

Making Connections in Music Therapy

Claire Flower

People who live on continents get into the habit of regarding the ocean as journey's end... For people who live on islands the sea is always the beginning. (Jonathan Raban 1987, p.299)

Introduction

This chapter is about journeys in music therapy. It is about my journey and the ways in which my thinking and practice have developed. Having had two children in the last three years, I have sometimes felt like an islander myself, cut off from the mainland of music therapy. This distance, and the experience of motherhood, have given me an opportunity to think again about my own clinical approach. In particular, I have had to think again about my place in the lively debate about where the meaning in music therapy lies, whether in the music itself or in the words which describe it.

There are strong voices on either side of the discussion. For example, in a recent *British Journal of Music Therapy* article, Ruth Walsh makes striking use of verbal material in her work with an adolescent girl with learning disabilities (Walsh 1997). She voices a widespread but nonetheless controversial view. It is, she believes, rarely enough to leave an understanding of what is going on implicit in the music alone. Similar arguments have been put forward by Mary Priestley (1994) when she proposes that for any musical shift or significant moment to be understood fully, it must be processed verbally.

Therapists such as Gary Ansdell (1995) take a phenomenological approach and believe that the work needs no verbal accounts. The music can, as he puts it, 'mean itself' (p.30). The therapist's musical response to a client constitutes an intrinsic interpretation, one contained within the musical relationship.

These approaches, the more verbal and the purely musical, can often become quite polarized. It does seem, though, that there is a substantial middle ground. Sandra Brown (1998) explores the question of how much change in the work with one child was brought about by a focus on the musical interaction and how much by attention to the symbolic and non-musical.

With regard to this, it is interesting to look at the work of one British music therapist who is also a child psychotherapist. Margaret Hughes (1996) describes how, in working with one autistic child, it was important, as well as working verbally, to think musically about the sounds the child was making. The child was able to integrate fragmented aspects of himself through the sounds he made and the imitating responses of the therapist. At some points in the therapy, Hughes found that he could be reached through this musical approach more readily than through words.

Annie Eppe (1998), working in Belgium, also seems to try to hold the middle ground with her concept of 'Dual Listening'. Here attention is given to the content – that is, the physical, musical and verbal expression of the client – and the form of the therapeutic relationship. In some of the work she describes, the musical and the psychodynamic are held in mind simultaneously. At other times there appear to be phases in which either the psychodynamic or the musical have prominence. An example of this would be the working through of an ending in a therapeutic group which culminates in the creation of a choir.

It has, perhaps, been a crisis of confidence in our own musical approach that has seen many music therapists working increasingly through words. In my own work, even though I work primarily within a framework of creative improvisation, there have been periods in which words have eclipsed the music. This has been truer with some clients than with others. My supervision has also come from music therapists training as psychotherapists, and this has exerted its own inevitable influence.

But, in the period of the last year, I have found myself returning to my musical roots, wanting to reassess my use of improvisation, how I listen and how I respond. Perhaps motherhood has strengthened in me the capacity to communicate without words. In this chapter I am presenting work with two boys, who are both, for differing reasons, without spoken language.

In this work, as in much of my practice, the focus of the work lies in the music, but the thinking is not solely about the music. Improvising with a child makes different levels of thinking possible. For instance, I can think clearly about the music itself, analysing the component features carefully, but I may also contemplate the musical experience – how it feels to improvise with this child and what the child's understanding of his or her own music may be. Within the space created by improvising together, I try to consider the nature of the child's internal world and the interpersonal connection made with me, looking particularly at how these two areas are reflected and developed in the music.

Clinical material

Steven and Nathan are two boys with differing problems. Steven is nine years old and has cerebral palsy. He can hardly move and has no speech. He does understand much that is said and, despite his difficulties, gives the impression of considerable emotional maturity.

Nathan is seven. He presents a stark contrast to Steven, being physically strong and agile but with far less understanding of himself or his world. His general developmental delay is compounded by his severe language and communication difficulties.

At the time of writing, both boys have received music therapy for one year. In each case the sessions have been co-worked, with myself at the piano and Rosie Monaghan, another music therapist, acting as co-therapist. As will become apparent, her role has differed with each child.

Case study 1: Steven

Steven is an alert, amiable boy, to a large extent imprisoned by his body. It is thought that Steven's understanding of language is good and staff working with him have been exploring ways of helping him to express himself more fully. They have attempted to use his eye-pointing in conjunction with yes and no cards but have found him, until recently, unable or unwilling to use them. He would often look away, seeming to choose not to respond. Staff found this very difficult to deal with and it was partly out of their frustration that he was referred to music therapy.

Starting to work with Steven was unsettling. His disabilities seemed overwhelming to me, and his physical state precarious. My main aim was simply to create a relaxed, musical environment into which Steven could come as he was able. How, I wondered, would he respond to the music? Would he be able to make his own sounds, what would they be like? Was using the instruments possible and, if so, how? Most of all, I wondered if there could be any points of contact between us.

Ansdell (1995) describes the importance of an initial experience of musical contact as a precursor to further, more complex musical meetings. He describes contact as happening when 'the client hears himself being heard' (p.71). I understand this as arising when the client realizes that my improvisation is an attempt to incorporate what they are doing and respond to it. It seemed, from moments in those early sessions, as though Steven not just heard himself being heard but was not at all surprised by the experience. He seemed highly motivated to engage in the musical relationship and prepared to use whatever means he could to achieve that.

For example, at the beginning of a session early on in our work together I began a gentle, improvisation on arpeggios around A major, looking for a response. The responses were small but distinct. Steven's head came up, his eyes searched for mine, then followed my hands on the keys. When I left a slight pause, he came in clearly with a beautifully placed vocal phrase, B–C sharp, picking up the tonality of my playing. As a tentative 'hello' emerged from his initiative, he reached forward with his right hand towards the keyboard.

The task in this period, and still now to some extent, was to refine our listening and watching to catch the more subtle nuances of Steven's movements, sounds and breaths. It was easy to become hooked into the 'can't dos' of Steven's world. Steven can't keep his head up, Steven can't eye point consistently, Steven has poor use of his arms. In fact, Steven began to show us the range of his 'can dos', which were actually many and varied. They were just within a smaller scale than we were used to seeing.

As the potential for musical meeting became clearer, we explored two main channels of communication: Steven's use of voice and of piano.

Looking first at the vocal material, his pitch range is small, roughly a perfect fifth from E above middle C to the A below. His sounds are often soft but usually distinct and becoming more so as Steven experiments with a wider range of sounds. Many of his sung sounds come from an out breath, a sighed 'hey...'. This has quite naturally been worked into singing 'hello'. The range of other single consonant or vowel sounds has grown, sometimes with a number of syllables strung together. Although Steven often becomes tense at other times when using his voice, both his mother and speech therapist have commented on how relaxed and free Steven has seemed to be while vocalizing in music therapy.

Given the musical space, Steven has been able to initiate and sustain periods of vocal dialogue. This became more evident approximately six months into our work. In one particular instance, Steven's slight agitation at the start of the session was reflected by a semitonal clash in my music – nothing too discordant, just the feeling of there being a slight edge to our meeting, and to his state today. Maybe that edge is reflected too in the music being more staccato, less pedalled, and having, at least at the beginning, no harmonic filling. After a minute, in which Steven has been moving his mouth, as though readying himself to make a sound, a pause in the music allows him the space he needs to come in.

A period of vocal turn taking follows, which is sustained for more than a minute. The music is sparked by a falling minor third phrase which Steven initiates and which we both continue. As I provide a staccato harmonic accompaniment, the short melodic phrases are passed between us, sometimes in their original form, sometimes inverted. The vocal dialogue is striking in its pace and quality. In my mind I compare it with a typical spoken interaction with Steven. Here the pace would be slow and the quality limited by Steven's reliance on yes and no answers. By contrast, this vocal exchange was built largely on his own initiatives and could move at a quicker, livelier tempo than any other form of interaction.

This includes interaction at the piano, Steven's other area of focus. Sitting at the top end of the piano, Steven can reach out to the keyboard. Sometimes he can strike a single key, his hand staying there until he pulls it off to reorganize himself. More often, though, his arm will come down in a great sweep, creating descending clusters of sound. At this point in the work I often reflect these quite directly in my music, using similar shapes and harmonies to give not a direct imitation but a general impression of his sounds.

Quite unexpectedly, in one session, it struck me just how much of our music had a downward pull to it, predominantly because of the way in which Steven was able to play. I suddenly realized that we seemed stuck in our separate registers and that I could move up the keyboard towards him. Near the end of the session I did just that.

Thinking about it later, it occurred to me that this downward pull, this feeling of falling, pervaded not just our music but also much of Steven's experience of life. It was a constant effort to keep his head upright and, without the shoulder straps on his chair supporting him, his upper body would fall forwards. He could raise his arm but it would then fall uncontrolled. The music which he produced was directly connected to his experience of living within an unruly body.

Through the music we had created, a striking musical depiction of Steven had emerged. Dominant themes were the downward spread clusters from Steven's right hand and the sighing vocalizations. Not moving from our distinct halves of the keyboard had left me in the murky depths, the music lacking any brightness or clarity. The slow pulse and the rather thick, pedalled texture left little space. What kind of musical picture was being painted here?

The concept of improvisation portraying an individual's experience, through sound, of 'himself-in-the-world' is described by Pavlicevic (1997). I wondered if our music was reflecting at least one important aspect of how it was to be Steven. Maybe we had concentrated on the floppy, falling aspects of Steven, those aspects particularly determined by his physical condition.

Within that particular session, my actions had been intuitive. In the simple act of crossing Steven's hands, a playful response had been elicited from him and a further connection made between us.

I was interested, though, to think about my intuitive response. What had occurred to cause me to think of the fallingness and to challenge it by crossing hands? Why had the thought not occurred to me before? Was it that I was not in tune with Steven or was it that the relationship was not yet ripe for a move on to the next stage?

I saw something similar happening in my younger daughter's world at the same time. Playing with her one day, she reached up to my face and I began a game of 'Where's Mummy's nose? Here it is', pointing and naming parts of my face as I did so. She looked quite bemused, although she seemed to enjoy the rhythm and energy of the game. Thinking about it afterwards, I wondered what had made me introduce the whole new concept of naming and pointing. Was she ready for it and, if so, how had I known that?

The next day, playing again, she seemed to remember it, reaching up for my face. As I said 'Where's Mummy's nose?', she hit it, right on the button, to great glee from Mum and big sister! A new game was born, with endless possibilities and variations.

To me, it felt similar to what was happening with Steven. We had made an initial connection and developed it to a point where something of a plateau had been reached. Then came a thought in my mind which sparked new musical and interpersonal possibilities: How can we understand the process at work here?

Vygotsky's (1978) concept of the proximal zone, as described by David Aldridge (1996) was helpful to me. The proximal zone is the area between what the child can do on their own and what they can do with the help of an adult. In terms of the play with my daughter, it meant taking the already acquired act of pointing one step further by naming what she was pointing at and expecting her to respond.

Aldridge believes this has significance for therapeutic work. He writes: 'The proximal zone, where child and therapist play together, awakening a potential and extending the possibilities for the child, appears to be an important concept for music therapy and is critical in achieving new creative possibilities in the therapeutic relationship' (p.247).

It has been helpful to think of this on two levels. First, that of 'new creative possibilities'. Musically, there were obvious ways that this could happen. The texture could lighten by changing registers, but also by lifting the sustaining pedal. Melodic lines could change direction, lifting the music and, interestingly, often at the same time, seeming to assist Steven in lifting his head and shoulders. Second, I could think about the ways in which those new possibilities might lead to changes in the relationship. Perhaps these new musical ideas could help portray Steven as he might be in the world, exploring often overlooked or not yet discovered aspects of himself. Here is a nine-year-old boy who is often thought of as being fragile and in need of protection and security. Maybe there is in him a greater robustness and the potential to develop this quality further. I wondered what would happen if, musically, he were teased or challenged a little. What new connections would that bring both within himself and between us?

A few sessions later a small incident gave at least a hint of an answer. Vocalizing together at the piano, I inadvertently landed on a chord too heavily. Steven jumped violently, his whole body lurching to one side in his chair. A moment of panic for me but, after only an instant of hesitation, Steven smiled and the joke was born. At an earlier stage in our work I may have worried about him being too fragile for this but he not just tolerated but actually enjoyed it, giggling as I repeated the 'mistake'. Rather like a wrong note in an improvisation which leads in a totally new direction, this accidental happening, which jarred slightly, seemed to enlarge the potential for Steven and I to grow.

A key issue in the growth of the relationship has been to do with waiting and listening closely. At times, waiting for Steven has been excruciating and at no time more difficult than in a session nine months into the work. Our improvisation had had a Prokofiev-like feel to it, quite jagged, with meandering chromatic lines. The music slowed, perhaps with a feeling that we had lost our contact, and I posed the musical question with a rising line: 'Where do we go from here?' In the long silence which followed, over a minute in length, my hands were held up, poised ready to play again. It was only as I eventually lowered my hands, however, wondering if, in fact, we had reached a conclusion, that Steven raised his hand and played a single note. My echoing of his single note an octave lower brought a wry smile to Steven's face.

At times, then, I have been able to wait, but at other times I have been aware of being too busy, of swamping Steven with a kind of musical 'mush'. It has been painful to come out of some recent sessions feeling frustrated by my musical part in them and feeling strongly a sense of failing Steven.

But, as always, there are different levels at which I need to think about this. There are very practical things I can do, musically, to make a better context for Steven. I can refresh my improvisation skills, practice playing without my foot being glued to the sustaining pedal and think about excursions into other areas of tonality.

But something valuable is in danger of being lost if I approach this too quickly. Being faced with this musical dilemma may actually be a part of the present connection with Steven, informing me about our relationship now and my experience of him. I feel limited by my playing, frustrated, unable to do what I know in my head I would like to do. Maybe the feeling is not mine alone. Is this something of what it is like to be Steven, to have the urge and the clear intent to communicate but to be frustrated in the carrying out of that intent? If I feel limited, that can only be a fraction of the constraint which he feels.

In some ways, then, it is no surprise that my response is often to be 'doing' something, to fill the space left by the nodding head, the unruly arm. Perhaps, in my being busy and musically active, we none of us have to feel the reality of Steven's disability. To see how little he can do can be very painful. His capacity to make connections with the world around and the people in it can seem so limited. Yet, in music, and the richness of the musical relationship, he continually shows the wish to make those connections and the longing to be as fully Steven as possible.

Case study 2: Nathan

A sharp contrast to the very limited physical movement possible for Steven is seen in the almost perpetual motion of Nathan, a seven-year-old child with a complex diagnostic picture of developmental delay. My initial impressions of Nathan were of a breathtakingly energetic child who raced around the music therapy room as though a coiled spring within him has suddenly been released. Backwards and forwards he ran, slapping each surface he encountered, then clapping loudly or slapping his thighs.

His frantic ranging around the room and bouncing from the walls seemed not so much an attempt to get out as an effort to work out where the boundaries were. Where did he begin and end? What was wall, drum, floor and what was 'him'? He seemed utterly bewildered.

He was unable to sit down or stay in one place to play, so Rosie, the co-therapist, held out a large tambour, trying to 'catch' him as he circumnavigated the room time after time. Sometimes his playing would consist of a slap as he passed by. If he paused, with arms outstretched and hands held rigidly, he would execute a large rocking movement, hitting the instrument. For many sessions he could only play a single beat for each rock before rushing back to the wall. It was difficult to make any musical contact and almost impossible to feel as though he had any sense of hearing himself or of being heard by us.

At this point in the work I was struck that my music with Nathan seemed to have no sense of depicting Nathan as 'himself-in-the-world'. The music was solid and simple. Surely music portraying Nathan should be far more chaotic and discordant? Why would I do one thing for Steven and another with Nathan?

Pavlicevic (1997) emphasizes that it is only when an interpersonal contact has been made that it is really possible to offer a portrayal in sound of our clients. That happened relatively easily with Steven, but it felt, at this point, as though no such contact had yet been made with Nathan. Perhaps, in this session, my music reflected more the urgency of providing structure and boundaries, creating a solid musical space in which we might connect. Was the task at the moment more intrapersonal, helping Nathan to make sense of the room and his body within that room before he could make any further connections with us?

Daniel Stern (1985) talks about the baby using its body as a reference point through which to understand its diverse experiences. Nathan's very physical way of being in music therapy seemed to echo that stage. For example, looking at the drum but also feeling it and, often, licking it too. He seemed to use all his senses to understand the environment and himself within it.

Simple musical structures seemed best suited to this task – structures with short phrases, frequent repetition and simple, grounded harmonies. Our 'hello' song, for example, had a very basic structure in 2/2, picking up on Nathan's gross rocking movement and emphasizing the minim.

This large movement seemed to be the point at which a musical contact could be made. We were unsure whether he 'heard' his own movement and beating through our improvisation but he certainly began to extend his playing. Fairly quickly, he moved from only hitting the drum once before running off to playing for maybe 2, 3 or 4 beats. It felt as though he was beginning to organize his experiences into more meaningful units. Maybe he was even beginning to string those units together.

At that moment, though, he seemed to have no means of dividing his minim beat. In contrast to his speed around the room, his playing was heavy and laborious. His hand movements seemed so intrinsically linked to his whole body movement that his hands didn't seem able to work independently. This unrefined use of his limbs and hands limited his capacity to move on musically. It seemed to arise not out of any physical difficulty but out of some internal connection to himself that was lacking.

In a session five months after starting music therapy, Nathan did show the capacity to change in this respect. For the first time, he divided the beat and used two crotchets quite accurately as we sang his name. I want to focus in more depth on this important session as Nathan's achievement in subdividing the beat seemed to herald the beginning of a different feeling in the room.

Nathan continued to be quite mobile but seemed somehow less committed to his racing around, as though searching for an alternative. That alternative seemed to come when Nathan began a clear sequence of play. Periods of quiet, intimate play near the drum were followed by episodes of flight around the room. There were four periods of play in all, which grew longer following each episode of flight.

The whole sequence was initiated by Nathan, who, in the first of the four periods, knelt briefly beside the drum. He moved away for a time, then, in the second episode of play, bent down on all fours at the side of the drum, with a clear smile and unspoken invitation to Rosie. She moved with him, matching many of his movements. Nathan slowly and carefully pulled at his fingers, looking intently at them as though seeing them for the first time.

There are a number of significant changes here. The pace altered, as Nathan unusually remained still for a time. I noticed the change in his position too. Instead of being upright and trying to climb, or prone but with his face hidden away, he could be on the floor but in an open working position. The change in dynamics, to something other than forte, was striking too.

Maybe most importantly, it felt different in the room. Nathan's urge to draw another person into play was striking. He seemed able to share both a focus of attention (the drum) and even a feeling about what was happening. Did he have a sense that it was possible to share his experience with another?

Stern's (1985) view is that the sharing of subjective experiences is only possible when the infant can sense that others may experience a similar internal state to their own at that time. In pulling Rosie into his play in a slightly conspiratorial way, this was the first time I had felt that such a sharing of experiences was possible with Nathan.

In the next two episodes of play, the music changed. The minor key, together with the soft, staccato accompaniment, reflected the slightly uncertain, mysterious air. Nathan gazed at Rosie as they shared the drum. In the final section of play, he rested his hands, palms upwards, on the drum, allowing Rosie to tap them gently as we sang 'Here's my hand... Playing on the drum with my hand'.

This was, and is now, so exciting. Nathan's statement of special educational needs described a boy with a 'fleeting attention span...oblivious to those around him...who shows no signs of purposeful play or meaningful interaction with his environment'. Now we saw him beginning to connect both with his environment and with those around him.

These connections were to be further strengthened. In a subsequent session, having played together at the large drum, Nathan clearly looked first at Rosie and then at the tambour propped against the cupboard. He moved swiftly towards it, picked it up and handed it, with a half-smile, to Rosie. As she took it and held it out for him, he began to play.

This important moment echoes Trevarthen and colleagues' (1997) concept of secondary intersubjectivity. They describe the infant as beginning to point and gesture, increasingly interested in sharing their world and the objects within it. In Nathan's case this was different to any previous sharing. The initiative did not come from Rosie trying to tempt Nathan into playing.

This was Nathan, seeing the tambour, seeing Rosie, and making a connection between the three elements, delighting himself and us in the process.

Having worked more closely with Rosie, Nathan has lately shown an interest in connecting more directly with me. More and more of our work has taken place over the top of the piano, Nathan leaning over to engage. He often seems very alive, his eyes alive and searching, his face responsive.

At times, I have been particularly interested in the more subtle means by which he can now regulate the intensity of his interactions, an important developmental achievement (Stern 1985). In the past he had taken flight. Now, resting his elbows on the piano, he might hide his face with his hands but then bursts out, seeming to enjoy the continued contact. He backs away from Rosie at the drum but maintains the eye contact throughout.

Now, too, we have moved away from the heavy rocking music which characterized so much of the earlier music. The simple grounded musical structures with which we started have given way to a more spare, dissonant style. This seems to connect more directly with Nathan's movements and sounds. Now the music does seem to give a fuller portrayal of Nathan as himself in the world.

This did not seem possible earlier because of the necessity to create boundaries and structures through the music. In making an initial contact it had seemed helpful to mark Nathan's rocking movements strongly, often placing the downbeat on the stamp of his foot or the beat of his hand. It had served a purpose in helping Nathan to hear himself. Now that a new level of interpersonal connection was possible, to continue with that emphasis seemed limiting. It is only now that I can think with any clarity about the broader significance of the way we have played at different stages of the work. It is only now that the music between us has a feeling of life.

Conclusion

When I was starting to write this chapter, I was caught up in the middle of a gripping novel: *Snow Falling on Cedars* (Guterson 1995). The author succinctly describes the dilemma of the inhabitants of the island on which the story is set:

Islanders were required by the very nature of their landscape to watch their step moment by moment. No one trod easily upon the emotions of another ... They could not speak freely because they were cornered;

everywhere they turned there was water and more water, a limitless expanse of it in which to drown. They held their breath and walked with care. (p.385)

In some ways, both Steven and Nathan can be seen as islanders, cornered and with a limitless expanse of water in which to drown. Steven's physical disabilities and isolation threaten to overwhelm him. Nathan, too, seems at risk of drowning in a sea of unintegrated experiences of himself and other people.

Our task in the work has been to jointly construct a causeway which links island and mainland. For all the complexity of this task, the lessons themselves are very simple. I have had to learn to listen more acutely, attending to the most minute communications. It has been necessary to reflect on both musical and non-musical gestures and the nuances of my own responses, musical and otherwise. I have had to think about what all this information tells me about the internal worlds of Steven and Nathan, and what can be understood about their relationships with Rosie and I. This process of listening to and thinking about our sessions has often revealed the new seeds which are trying to grow. These, in turn, have needed to be planted in the music itself.

This emphasis on the music has been the dominant theme of the last year of my work. Since qualifying, many models have been helpful to me in learning to think about therapeutic work. They have also, sometimes, been undermining, emphasizing ways of working in which I have not been trained. So, for example, I may find myself feeling that I ought to be working in the style of a child psychotherapist. When I do this, it feels like an impersonation, not really me. For me, as a clinician, there can be a terrible deadness to this feeling, which directly affects the quality of any therapeutic work which can be done. The simple fact has been that I myself have felt more alive and authentic working in and thinking about the music. This, after all, is what I have been trained to do.

It is a dilemma which does not seem to be mine alone. When working with music therapy trainees, I have been struck by the fact that some, who have powerful analytic thinking, struggle to work effectively in the music. Others, who work skilfully in the music, sometimes lack the capacity to think therapeutically about what might be going on. These can easily be blind spots in the training that we provide. Holding both these strands seems to be one of the challenges for our profession.

Keeping the music at the forefront of the work is important, not just for ourselves and for our clients but for our colleagues in other professions. The musical interaction is direct and powerful, generating both information and opportunities for change. This is increasingly recognized by our colleagues from other disciplines. While much emphasis is on how we can apply other ways of thinking to music therapy, I want to stress the importance of music therapists giving their particular input into the wider professional environment. We need to learn to talk to non-musicians about the music our clients make and the information it gives us about their worlds.

Music therapy can be an integrated part of professional practice. In the recent book *Children with Autism*, the chapter by Jacqui Robarts on music therapy demonstrates how we can also play a part in wider professional thinking (Trevarthen *et al.* 1997). All of this involves music therapists recognizing that connections need to be built between our particular island and the worlds of other associated professionals. David Aldridge (1996) vividly describes us as a profession in the process of building these and other important bridges. When these connections are not present, the work can be undermined. When they are present, the container available to our clients is strengthened and the power of the work that can take place within it is enhanced.

This chapter has principally been about the bridges built in the work with Steven and Nathan. It has been about connections tentatively or firmly made. I am grateful to Steven and Nathan for allowing me to be a part of those connections, and to their families for allowing me to write about them. As the work continues, I feel excited and moved by the potential for it to change and grow.

Acknowledgements
I would like to acknowledge my gratitude to Esme Towse, Margaret Hughes and Sandra Brown, who have all, at different times, supervised my work and helped it grow. Rosie Monaghan features in these case studies as my co-therapist and much of the thinking about this work has been shared between us in a way that has been rewarding and very enjoyable. Lastly, for all his support and wise thoughts, many thanks to Steve.

Glossary

Phenomenological: a phenomenological approach to music therapy is one in which the therapist seeks to think about, and work with, the client's musical material without offering further interpretation.

Proximal Zone: the distance between what a child can do on their own, particularly in this instance, in music therapy, and what they have the potential for doing when playing together with the therapist.

Secondary intersubjectivity: as described by Trevarthen, the process by which the infant seeks to share experiences with others by shifting attention from objects to people and back again. Also described as person–person–object interaction.

References

Aldridge, D. (1996) *Music Therapy Research and Practice in Medicine.* London: Jessica Kingsley Publishers.

Ansdell, G. (1995) *Music for Life.* London: Jessica Kingsley Publishers.

Brown, S. (1998) *The Music, the Meaning, and the Therapist's Dilemma.* Paper presented at the 4th European Music Therapy Congress, Leuven, Belgium.

Eppe, A. (1998) *Dual Listening.* Paper presented at the 4th European Music Therapy Congress, Leuven, Belgium.

Guterson, D. (1995) *Snow Falling on Cedars.* London: Bloomsbury.

Hughes, M. (1996) *The Use and Function of Sound Towards the Development of a Sense of Body-Ego.* Unpublished child psychotherapy qualifying paper. London: Tavistock Clinic.

Pavlicevic, M. (1997) *Music Therapy in Context.* London: Jessica Kingsley Publishers.

Priestley, M. (1994) *Essays on Analytical Music Therapy.* Philadelphia: Barcelona Publishers.

Raban, J. (1987) *Coasting.* London: Picador.

Stern, D. (1985) *The Interpersonal World of the Infant.* New York: Basic Books.

Trevarthen, C., Aitken, K., Despina, P. and Robarts, J. (1997) *Children with Autism.* London: Jessica Kingsley Publishers.

Vyptosky, L. (1978) *Mind in Society.* Cambridge, MA: Harvard University Press.

Walsh, R. (1997) 'When having means losing: Music therapy with a young adolescent with a learning disability and emotional and behavioural difficulties.' *British Journal of Music Therapy 11,* 1.

CHAPTER 7

Client-Centred Music Therapy for Emotionally Disturbed Teenagers Having Moderate Learning Disability

John Strange

The setting

Under the English educational system, pupils with a wide range of problems and pathologies are broadly described as having 'learning difficulties'. Using the DSM-IV classification (American Psychiatric Association 1993), the majority would be said to suffer mild to profound mental retardation, but many also have other disorders first diagnosed in infancy, childhood or adolescence. Also found are disorders from many other DSM-IV categories, which either cause or aggravate learning difficulties or are themselves caused by the stresses associated with learning difficulties.

Theoretical orientation

The varied client needs I have encountered have led me to adopt a corresponding variety of approaches. Sometimes I have given co-improvised music a much less central role than it plays in the work of Nordoff and Robbins (1977) which first attracted me to the profession. As the three cases discussed below illustrate, I have learned to take account of how each client is prepared to work with me. All three have only moderate mental retardation and were referred to music therapy because of additional problems, as described in the case material.

I have borrowed the term 'client-centred therapy' for this work from the approach described by Rogers (1961) because each of these three clients and I together negotiated ways of working congruent with their own views of the world and of their needs, rather than my imposing on them a particular framework or approach. Beyond that important resemblance, the parallel with Rogers is far from exact. Indeed, it is doubtful whether a music therapy approach should be too closely modelled upon one designed for use in predominantly verbal therapy.

A psychoanalyst might view the resistances which emerge in clients' therapy as signs of unconscious fears and conflicts, which it is essential to address. I prefer, by contrast, to consider what such areas of resistance may tell me of unconscious forces but then to work round, rather than through, them. It is important not to precipitate a withdrawal from therapy. Many clients have already experienced rejection and have difficulties which increase the likelihood of further rejection. To insist on a way of working which these clients find threatening can endanger the whole therapeutic relationship.

I tried to maintain 'unconditional positive regard' (Rogers 1961) for these clients, without giving the glib praise so frequently used in special education to motivate effort and reinforce every achievement. I hoped that musical events and experiences would provide their own intrinsic motivation. Few clients in special education have any concept of therapy as a resource for self-development and the relief of distress, though the first client I shall discuss did intuitively realize this aspect of the work. Most, however, have experienced the musical activities that have been widely, and not always intelligently, used for a multitude of purposes throughout special education. The more intensive and focused use of music as therapy affects clients in various ways. Sometimes rebellion emerges strongly as a theme but the work with Norman, Donald and Laura (not their real names) was dominated, for me, by the recognition of their underlying anxiety.

Case study 1: Norman

Norman was referred at the age of fifteen with a diagnosis of moderate learning disability of unknown aetiology. Teaching staff felt his educational progress was being hampered by anxiety. He had suffered a brief incident of sexual abuse when he was ten. At the age of thirteen he moved from a country town to a London suburb and a new school.

Soon after I started work with him, Norman's emotional vulnerability became evident. A female student confronted him with the news that another student had just attempted to rape her in a public toilet. For many weeks, Norman felt a mixture of horror and guilt towards the perpetrator and had difficulty in separating reality from disturbing delusions. He was given psychological counselling, and if he spoke of his concerns in the music therapy sessions, I remained as a neutral listener. I saw my role as helping him to regain his confidence and the ability to tolerate reasonable levels of anxiety.

In his first session Norman immediately chose a cabasa and started to play. He did so continuously for three sessions. For months he played only this and other small unpitched percussion instruments, explaining to me that he found larger instruments strange. In a typical session he would start cautiously. Gradually, the amorphous rhythms would become more regular, forming an almost featureless monotony. The basic beat might undergo some patterned division but no one rhythm became obsessive. Contrasts of detail arose from occasional experiments with different ways of holding the instruments but these did not lead to changes of mood. His facial expression remained blank, with his eyes fixed on the instrument.

I judged that the inexpressive quality of Norman's playing was specific to the therapy situation, rather than pathological. Perhaps playing an instrument in a one-to-one situation placed him in an exposed position in which it was unsafe to show emotion and yet necessary to comply with imagined adult expectations by playing continuously until given permission to stop. I had observed that there were situations, in the classroom and outside with friends, when his behaviour and manner were relatively extrovert.

Feeling that for Norman's playing to develop it needed to be supported rather than challenged, I accompanied him on the piano or, occasionally, other percussion instruments. He said that he preferred me to use the piano but gave no reason. In my playing I tried to confirm, by reflection, the general mood and style of his playing whilst providing a gentle sense of forward progress. I also added, unobtrusively, varied accompaniments to reduce the monotony which I judged was not intentional but the result of his overcautious approach. I tried not to introduce strongly contrasted material which might have been experienced as directive, or even dismissive of what he was offering.

For some months he would take any gap in the piano part as a signal to stop. Gradually, he became able to accept short and predictable breaks in my playing without stopping himself, but he did not follow this example and punctuate his own playing. He found it difficult to end the music and relied on me to do this, although as soon as we had stopped playing at the end of

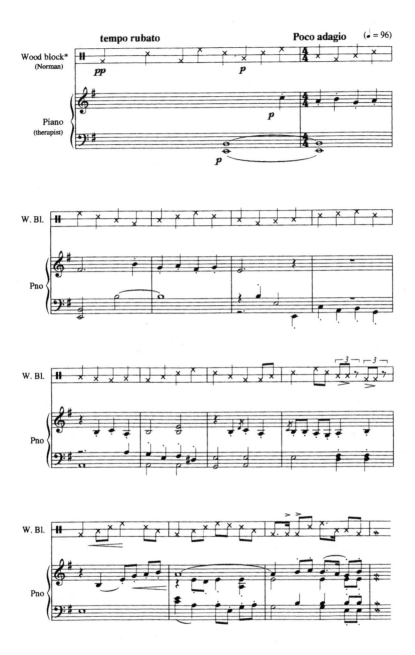

Figure 7.1
* The wood block only produced a single indefinite pitch but Norman struck it at different points, as shown by the positions of note heads.

the session he had no problem with leaving. His difficulty with ending the music could possibly have been interpreted to him as the result of past experiences of powerlessness, but I did not feel that to do so would have been helpful.

If Norman made any small change in his playing, I would slightly amplify it. The only way in which he ever seemed to imitate me was by briefly reflecting back some of the divisions I added to his basic rhythm. Although I was following him, he always said that it was he who was following me. I thought it likely that he considered that following was the most appropriate and safest role for him. Figure 7.1 shows the opening moments of improvisation from an early session and illustrates many of the above observations.

As the weeks passed, I felt weighed down by the emotional flatness of Norman's music. I began to feel he might be depressed as well as anxious. I did not wish to present an incongruous alternative of light-hearted music but I tried using varying levels of dissonance to hint at slightly contrasting moods which I wondered if he might like to explore. He gave no sign of noticing. Was he insensitive to harmony or purposely ignoring discords or modulations which could have suggested feelings he did not wish to admit to?

I became aware of the danger, when a client's music presents such a blank canvas, that the therapist, slipping into a sort of musical free association (rather as the Freudian analyst's self-concealment encourages a client to free associate verbally), may mistake the musical products of his own unconscious for those of the client.

Norman's current emotional state, as evident from the reports of other staff and his mother and also in his conversation walking to and from the session, seemed never to be reflected in his playing. After the disturbing incident described above, he gave up parts of several sessions to talking about his anxiety, but I could detect no change in his playing. There was thus no question of working directly with his anxieties through the music. Perhaps, having stood at the brink of psychosis, Norman sensed that such self-revelation would be too threatening, and this defence had to be respected.

Norman seemed to intuit that he needed to restore his own peace of mind. I now believe his bland, uneventful music was providing him with an inner calm amidst chaos, an anchor in stormy seas, a form of meditation to steady his emotions. Although starting to realize this at the time, I still sought a

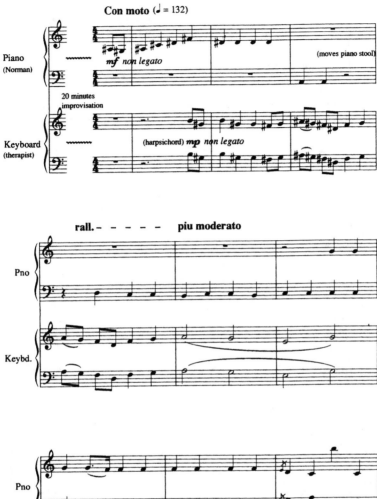

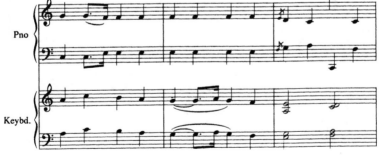

Figure 7.2

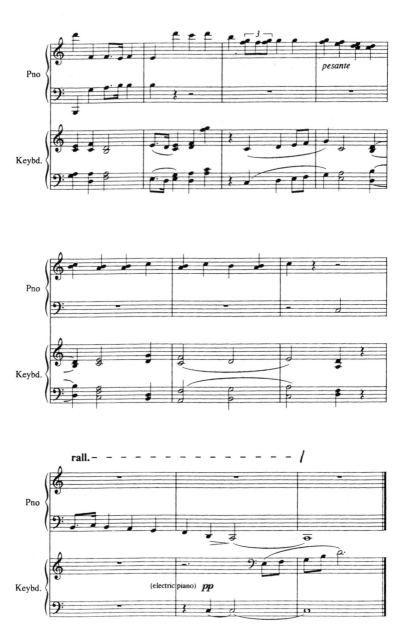

Figure 7.2 (continued)

more active role for myself in Norman's process of rehabilitation. If I could not induce him to express his painful feelings musically, perhaps I could desensitize him to threatening experiences by providing musical shocks which he could learn to assimilate. This was not effective. Norman demonstrated his absolute concentration on his own playing by totally ignoring the conflicting metres, dynamic jolts and sharp discords I tossed at him. Once, Norman told me that his playing in our sessions was peaceful and unlike anything else he did. By contrast, his own unaided efforts to use music for comfort consisted of listening to hard-rock music at maximum volume in his bedroom – more a case of blowing his mind than of focusing it.

After eight months of therapy, Norman was still only playing one small hand-held unpitched instrument per session, such as cabasa, woodblock or jingle, but his rhythms were at last gradually acquiring more variety and life. By now I knew he must be allowed to move at his own pace. Change must be a process of self-discovery, not the product of pressure from me. My musical support as accompanist, however, remained essential to this process as I highlighted and developed the clearer rhythmic motives and small dynamic contrasts he introduced. This musical equivalent of 'unconditional positive regard' was all Norman needed to maintain the confidence to proceed.

In the ninth month of therapy Norman moved to his first melodic instrument, a small glockenspiel. A few weeks later he moved to an electronic keyboard and a few weeks later, again, to the piano, which he had previously seen as my instrument. His playing gained steadily in rhythmic invention, liveliness of tempo and contrast of texture, exploiting the range of the keyboard and all the untutored agility of fingers and arms at his command. Figure 7.2 illustrates this change.

Around this time, Norman talked of an ambition to ban bull fighting, which, whilst not fully in touch with practicalities, indicated a more optimistic and proactive outlook than a few months earlier. His playing became more responsive to changes of rhythm and dynamics that I introduced, either by imitation or by responding with contrasting ideas of his own. It seemed that his music was at last secure enough not to require his undivided attention, so that he could now attend also to mine. This enabled him to adopt the contrasting calmer moods I occasionally offered from my quieter keyboard.

I felt the changes in Norman's music indicated a greater self-confidence and a letting go of defences which could restrict social intercourse. Therapy was concluded after eighteen months by mutual agreement and Norman maintained his emotional equilibrium and made good progress in his last year at school.

Case study 2: Donald

Donald was sixteen when I resumed the therapy he was reported to have started two years earlier with a previous music therapist shortly before the latter had left the school. Donald also had moderate learning disability of unknown aetiology. His main presenting problem in school was fairly frequent explosions of aggression, usually verbal, of a paranoid character.

Donald's ambition was to join the police force. He ignored the fact that his learning difficulty made this extremely unlikely. He was usually friendly, charming and humorous, respectful of adults and keenly interested in adult activities, attitudes and manners. The smallest threat to his self-esteem, however, could lead to an instant and quite startling temper tantrum directed against the offending pupil or staff member. His language and manner would become reminiscent of a drill-sergeant disciplining a new recruit.

The two groups most important to him were the church choir and the air cadet training corps. In the choir and in the corps he experienced being treated with dignity as an equal by others without learning disabilities. Both were highly disciplined groups where firmly enforced authority gave him security, protecting him not only from the provocations of others but also from losing his own self-control. His concept of an authority figure, however, seemed much harsher than he can have experienced in either choir or corps. Authority, to Donald, meant rigid control and instant punishment for the offender, and these traits surfaced in his own behaviour whenever he felt his dignity threatened. Donald wanted to spend his sessions listening to, and learning to play, military and church music, but the first five months of music therapy were shared with another pupil mainly interested in creating special effects on the electronic keyboard. So long as Donald felt secure in being fairly treated, he could show social skill and consideration for others and the two boys avoided serious disagreement. They would occasionally try to play together but usually worked independently at their separate interests, as though they could not actually hear each other's music.

I had initially hoped to establish free group improvisation, in which all three of us would listen and respond to each other's music. After five months it was clear that this goal was no nearer. A therapist trained in group analysis might have decided to explore this musical non-meeting as a symptom of social dysfunction but my solution was to ask the boys if they would prefer to be given individual sessions. Both were in favour.

Donald seized his chance for more individual attention, requesting an endless succession of military and church music. Sometimes he would ask me to write out the melodies of hymns or military marches, such as the 'Dambusters' theme, for him to play at home on a keyboard with numbered notes. Improvisation he utterly rejected, describing it as 'messing about'. Despite my distinctly un-authoritarian behaviour, Donald projected onto me some aspects of his concept of an authority figure. I was expected to be omnipotent, knowing and able to play every piece he requested. My occasional failures seemed to shock and disturb him. I felt like a jukebox, an inanimate dispenser of chosen tunes. If I demonstrated that I was an independent person, by improvising variations on his chosen tune, his condemnation could be as severe as that of the church authorities towards Bach's organ interludes in congregational chorales.

I felt concerned that I had nothing to offer Donald which might give him insight into his problems and enable him to gain control over his tendency to explode under stress. One day he told me that his throat was sore from 'putting people right'. I asked how he would feel if I were to 'put him right' by dictating the choice of music. He replied that this would be unfair. I gently pointed out that sometimes his instructions to me sounded like those of a dictator.

At this time the head teacher had recently retired and a successor had not yet been appointed. Donald told me that we must get one 'to keep people in order'. In his eyes, control was a vital necessity. When he requested Passiontide hymns, such as 'O Sacred Head, sore wounded', I drew his attention to the words describing Christ's suffering and non-violent resistance of evil, but he made plain his hatred of all such ideas.

When I suggested to Donald that he was only bringing part of himself to sessions and hiding his problems from me, he became agitated, humming and trying to distract me. A few weeks later, however, he did briefly share something painful with me – the funeral of a family member. He soon cut short my response, however, explaining that I 'might say something rotten'. The next week, after losing an argument with a member of staff, he tried to restore his self-respect by insisting on total control of every aspect of the session.

Before the summer break, feeling puzzled about how to proceed, I suggested that Donald should join a group of four in the autumn. I told him that equal time would be given to each member's choice of music or activity. He agreed to this, but as soon as the sessions started he tried to 'book' his share of the time, giving me details of how it should be spent, in advance of each session. I decided to offer him an additional twenty minutes on his own in the lunch hour, provided he stopped demanding special treatment in the group sessions. This was a clear boundary which I guaranteed to enforce and, therefore, appealed to Donald.

Thereafter, Donald became entirely co-operative, helpful, tolerant and aware of his companions' varying needs. One activity I suggested was that group members should think of someone else in the group, select an appropriate instrument and play in such a way that others could guess who was being described. He approached this potentially embarrassing game with humour rather than anxiety, poking fun at myself rather than at other students.

In group improvisations his contributions were more freely inventive than hitherto, using several percussion instruments previously neglected. He listened to others' music more than he had when with his original companion and was able to play a supporting rather than always a dominant role. He accompanied quietly and sensitively, as he had heard me doing, when a student with profound disabilities played. The only remnant of his obsession with discipline was his care over every detail of the 'rules' we had jointly agreed for certain activities. Most impressively, he never lost his temper over other pupils' inability to keep these 'rules'.

Donald was now coping with being one among equals, without a rigidly imposed external discipline. He still longed for individual attention but accepted that the place for this was his extra lunchtime session. Here his attitude remained egocentric, but I hoped he would be able to transfer the social responsibility evoked by the group music therapy experience into other situations with peers which required it. Therapy was terminated after two years when he left school.

Case study 3: Laura

Laura started work with me when she was thirteen-and-a-half. Psychological tests at five and six had revealed mild learning difficulties and low self-esteem likely to compound these over time. She also suffered from epilepsy and the drugs to control her complex partial seizures sometimes caused drowsiness. A major traumatic event involving violence within the family occurred when Laura was nine and the consequences still affect her

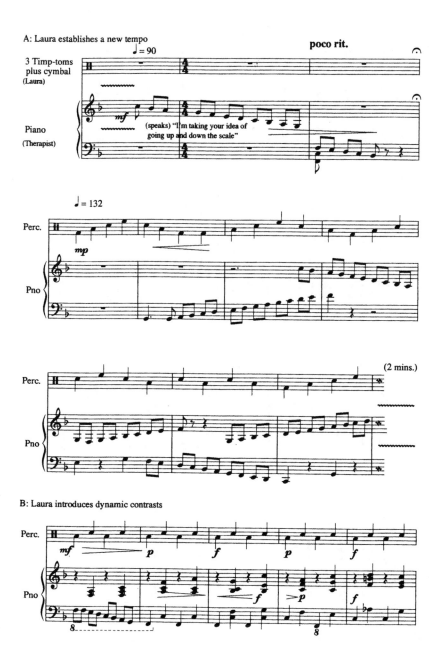

Figure 7.3

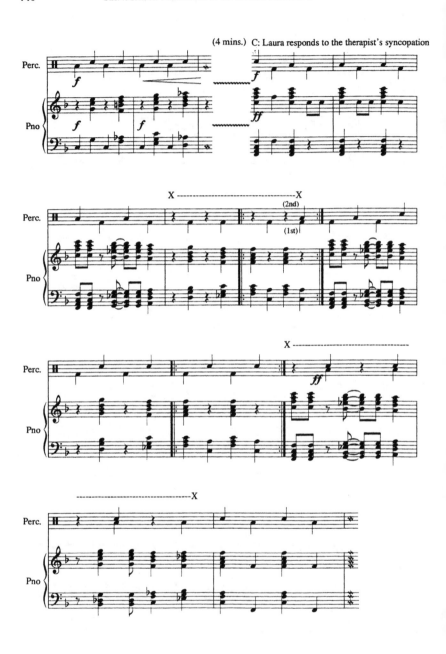

Figure 7.3 (continued)

domestic situation nine years later. At the age of eleven she spent many months in hospital suffering from myasthenia gravis. This has since been in remission but has left some neural impairment, chiefly to hands and mouth.

Laura had a paranoid concern with how others saw her, fed by a tendency to destroy valued friendships by taunting her friends over their failures and becoming violently aggressive in the face of even mild teasing. After assessing her, I decided that my aims would be to raise her self-esteem, improve motivation to counteract her lethargy and provide a musical channel for expressing painful and angry feelings.

For the first few months Laura spent parts of many sessions playing the drums and cymbal with a vigour surprising in someone generally so lethargic. Although limited by muscle weakness to simple rhythms in a moderate tempo, she showed a grasp of phrase structure and contrast, and even moments of mischievous humour. I followed and interacted with her from the piano in a flexible way such that, if she faltered, she need not feel she had 'gone wrong'. Figure 7.3 illustrates Laura's free improvisation on drums and cymbal.

I was hopeful that this bold, adventurous music making would boost Laura's confidence. Perhaps she might even feel ready soon to express some of her blacker moods in music and explore why she sometimes lost her temper and became violent with staff and other pupils.

Sadly, this phase did not last. After about six months it was clear that Laura wished to spend every session improving her keyboard playing. She constantly played a small selection of tunes which either someone had apparently taught her or she had invented herself. Whenever she hit a difficulty, she was eager for help, but the only kind she could make use of was an exact model she could imitate using her visual memory. This entailed using mostly my left hand, as she did, with minimal extension and no use of the thumb.

As soon as Laura was confident enough to play a small section of music without breaking down, I would accompany her on another keyboard. My reason for doing this was simple: without any accompaniment, the tunes she played sounded bare and, because of her uniformly heavy touch, crude. I judged that these were primarily defects of musical technique and that my accompaniment could complement her contribution, creating a more aesthetically pleasing total effect, which would also be more like what Laura had in mind when playing these tunes. This would, I hoped, motivate her to continue developing what abilities she had by making each small advance in learning the occasion for a pleasurable experience. Figure 7.4 illustrates a typical duet texture.

My goal for Laura was not musical attainment but an improvement in her low self-esteem as she realized that she could overcome difficulties and produce something that would command respect. As such activity was repeated month after month, however, I wondered how much I was really helping her. Laura still showed her low self-esteem by hitting her head when things went wrong, getting worse rather than better with each repeat of a problem passage and even blaming herself for my occasional mistakes.

I was also concerned that Laura's music seemed to bear little relation to the personality of the player. As soon as a piece was finally mastered, her playing of it sounded mechanical and all the tunes were relentlessly cheerful, despite her gloomy moods, seeming to deny all the paranoid and jealous feelings that threatened her relationships. I tried to address these instead by discussing problems that arose in the actual process of learning her tunes and only later drawing parallels with her social problems.

After three years of therapy Laura played the electric keyboard in front of the whole school. Though well prepared, she had an attack of stage fright. With my encouragement, and a very positive reception from the audience, she was able to complete the performance without a slip. This gave her concrete evidence to contradict her paranoid feeling before the performance that 'everybody is against me – they'll laugh at me'.

The following week Laura said that her hands felt weak. This led to a discussion of the effect of this on her playing. In the next session she talked about the acute phase of her myasthenia gravis and the disabilities with which it had left her. She still found it hard, however, to accept that other students, whom she finds annoying, also have disabilities and that these might explain some of their behaviour, although she did agree to stop bullying them in future. The following week I persuaded her to admit that my not criticizing her mistakes had helped her and suggested that she, in turn, should not criticize the mistakes of others. I also pointed out that her experience of embarrassment at being slow in learning music could help her understand when someone else was embarrassed. I felt Laura was now ready for the challenge of working with a peer in therapy and a student with Asperger's syndrome joined us. He had, by this time, largely overcome an earlier paranoia as debilitating as Laura's and was recognized in school as an exceptional guitar player, able to produce by ear convincing arrangements of almost any recorded music he heard. Far from being intimidated, Laura

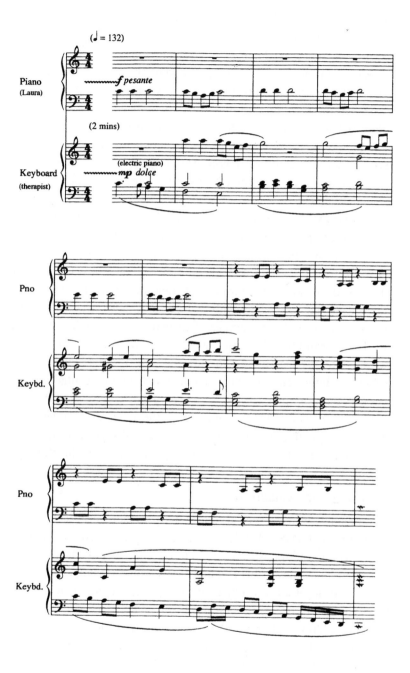

Figure 7.4

controlled her habit of self-criticism almost completely in his presence and allowed him to teach her part of 'Hello Dolly', a tune slightly harder than anything she had played before. She tolerated his lack of awareness of her difficulties and had the confidence to say when she wanted to stop. Relations between the two remained relaxed and I was sorry that after two months he decided to stop coming, pleading other commitments.

Shortly after this, Laura, for the first time, worked systematically at finding notes 'by ear' instead of relying on her mainly visual memory of their place on the keyboard. This involved singing as well as playing and, with much encouragement, she forced herself to hum back what I played, with growing accuracy.

Our discussions have covered her difficulty in curing a habitual mistake, factors which can make learning more stressful, the fact that everyone's achievement falls short of their efforts and dreams, and the problem of living in a world which does not understand or accept disability. I illustrated this last topic by making my normally flexible accompaniment to her tune suddenly mechanical and unyielding. Instead of subtly accommodating her unsteady tempo and her stumbles, I carried on as though not hearing. I hoped, by reminding her that she still needed me to allow for her imperfections, to encourage her to show the same flexibility towards others.

A lot of understanding has been achieved by an essentially cognitive approach, but this approach has only been possible because of the friendly relationship so painstakingly built up in the previous four years' music making. Recognizing that her own learning will always be slow, Laura now has the confidence to teach tunes to younger pupils in the lunch break.

Recording and evaluation

Music therapy given as a special educational provision must, according to the *Code of Practice* (HMSO 1994), have clearly stated objectives. The problem for a therapist adopting a client-centred approach is that to describe therapeutic outcomes in behavioural terms would prejudge the course of therapy. Instead of a list of objectives, therefore, I write down from two to four of the client's needs, as I perceive them, which I feel music therapy may be able to address. I then use these as headings, recording week by week under each heading the observations which relate to that need. I am then able to report, when required, the extent to which each need seems to have been met. Evaluation of the work has two facets, public and private. On the one hand, I have to report to parents and other professionals the progress each client is making. If there has been no corresponding progress in either educational achievement or relationships at home or school, this could raise questions about the value of a therapy whose benefits do not appear to have generalized, but, more often, the conclusion drawn is that music therapy has a particular relevance to the pupil as one area in which (s)he is making advances. Conversely, if comparable advances have been noted within and outside music therapy, I am careful not to claim a role for music therapy which I cannot substantiate, but it is gratifying how often others raise the possibility of such a causal relationship.

The other facet of evaluation is my own assessment of what has been achieved and where we are going, focusing more on my role and contribution. Observations scattered among my session notes may point to aspects of transference, as when Donald would regard even the mildest disagreement as my being a dictator, or countertransference, as when, in accompanying Norman's undemonstrative improvisations, I sensed the danger of attributing to him the feelings emerging in my own improvisation. Such conclusions would only be stated very obliquely, if at all, in written reports. Similarly, areas where I feel my strategies and music therapy techniques have been inept or inappropriate must be addressed but do not feature prominently in written reports.

The role of music

The cases of Norman, Donald and Laura illustrate how music can play a role very different from that which one first envisages. I hoped Norman's cautious and subdued improvisation would become more adventurous, but this did not even start to occur for many months. I also hoped he would be able to express through music some of his anxieties, but this only ever occurred verbally and he used music instead to express the steady centre of himself he wished to preserve. Eventually, through his own evolving musical expression, Norman came to see himself in a more positive light and strike out more assertively.

I hoped that the rigidity and harshness of Donald's rare keyboard improvisations, reminiscent of his autocratic behaviour, might become gentler and more flexible as a prelude to learning to let these aspects of his personality guide his behaviour. Instead, he chose to listen to, and sometimes learn to play, music with which he was already familiar and which reminded him of sources of authority upon which I felt he needed to become less dependent. He found his gentler, empathetic self only in the music he improvised in the second group, perhaps mainly through contact with those he perceived as more needy than himself.

I hoped Laura's confident, energetic and inventive drumming would become a foundation from which she could develop these attributes in other aspects of her life. I also hoped it would channel the anger that was being vented in aggressive outbursts. Instead, she persisted with her clumsy and inexpressive keyboard playing, forever being reminded of the inadequacy of her short-term memory, because only this seemed to her a socially valuable achievement. By overcoming obstacles, she attained a skill she could feel proud of. It was a risky process and, but for the understanding, warmth and enthusiasm of staff and pupils, when she eventually decided to play in assembly, her self-esteem could have been damaged rather than raised.

In each of these cases musical experiences led to some of the insights gained, and, equally important, music provided the framework and the motivation for developing a therapeutic relationship.

The role of the therapist

At the simplest level, I, as therapist, provided the opportunity for the developments described above to occur. Admittedly, I also attempted for a time to steer each client in directions he or she did not, in fact, choose to take. So my client-centred approach did not attain the sublimity of total detachment! But it was good enough — I was able, eventually, to accept and support unforeseen developments and these may have had a greater significance for the clients as they were treading paths they themselves had chosen.

As well as supporting their chosen uses of music, I offered a certain amount of normal person-to-person social interaction. I was careful to avoid a didactic or over-directive approach, but I did occasionally suggest possible lines of action, express agreement and disagreement, congratulate, commiserate, even tease — in fact, I did whatever I thought would create a relaxed atmosphere of mutual respect and trust without dependency.

Keeping the social interaction as natural and unremarkable as possible can help to reduce the strangeness some clients sense in the sudden musical freedom of the therapy session, after the directive approach of class music lessons. This was not a problem for Norman but Donald and Laura, both of whom had, in fact, shown themselves able to improvise and enjoy it, had acquired a fixed attitude that improvisation is just playing about and not real music. When socially they had become more trusting of me, they both gradually moved forward from this position to one where they might improvise if given a little encouragement.

What of the therapist's musical role? Musical skills such as acute listening and flexible and stylistic improvisation are not of use only in interactive music making. They were of equal value in providing a supportive but non-restricting accompaniment to Norman's improvisation. They enabled me to play Donald's favourite music by ear, either from memory or, occasionally, from tapes of band music that he brought. They allowed me to accompany Laura's stumbling tunes flexibly enough to keep in step and idiomatically enough (without ever eclipsing her part) to give both her and, eventually, her audience an impression that we were musically together. Music therapy, of whatever orientation, requires highly developed musical skills in the practitioner, although these need not necessarily focus on the keyboard.

Applications of the client-centred approach

Therapy involves change, and change can be stressful. Self-referred clients, voluntarily seeking therapy for problems of whose existence they are aware, are strongly motivated to change and, therefore, likely to continue attending when the experience proves stressful and puzzling. Clients such as school pupils who have been referred by others, on the other hand, may have no such motivation to change and, if free to leave (as I believe they should normally be), may do so if the experience proves too stressful.

To minimize this risk, the stresses involved should not be of a kind that clients are likely to perceive as imposed upon them by the therapist. One way to guard against this is to adopt a client-centred approach, in the sense of involving the client in all or most decisions as to how to proceed. Music therapy has the advantage of using an artistic medium which has some sort of significance, often at a deep level, for almost everyone. The three clients I have described were all sufficiently highly motivated by their existing attraction towards musical expression to attend therapy regularly.

Norman was already under severe emotional stress in the early months of therapy, and was additionally attending psychotherapy. Little, if anything, in the music therapy sessions exacerbated this. His need was not to relinquish maladaptive behaviours or thought patterns but to regain the sense of autonomy that his recent experiences had threatened. Donald and Laura, by contrast, sometimes displayed acutely antisocial behaviour. This may have been addressed rather obliquely in the therapy I have described but the process was not without stress – for example, Donald's extreme frustration when I first refused to carry out his instructions, or Laura's near defeat by stage fright and the first time we discussed the permanent nature of her disability.

In this client-centred approach the stresses of therapy feel to the clients like consequences of a process jointly negotiated with the therapist – a process which meets what they themselves perceive as their needs. A client-centred approach also provides a source of pride in achievement when clients feel that progress has been made along paths they themselves have chosen.

Glossary

Complex partial seizures: epileptic seizures in localized areas of the brain, causing disturbances of movement, sensation and behaviour but not complete loss of consciousness.

Myasthenia gravis: an autoimmune disease causing muscle weakness and fatigue, which worsen with exercise and improve with rest.

References

American Psychiatric Association (1993) *Diagnostic and Statistical Manual of Mental Disorders, Fourth Edition.* Washington DC: American Psychiatric Association.

HMSO (1994) *Code of Practice on the Identification and Assessment of Special Educational Needs.* London: Department for Education.

Nordoff, P. and Robbins, C. (1977) *Creative Music Therapy.* New York: John Day.

Rogers, C.R. (1961) *On Becoming a Person: A Therapist's View of Psychotherapy.* Boston: Houghton Mifflin.

CHAPTER 8

The Use of Creative Improvisation and Psychodynamic Insights in Music Therapy with an Abused Child

Pauline Etkin

The approach to music therapy that is at the heart of my work is that based on the teaching and research of Paul Nordoff and Clive Robbins (1971, 1977). Central to the approach is the use of music and clinical improvisation to establish a relationship with the client, provide a means of communication and self-expression, and effect change and the realization of potential. It is the belief in the music itself as the medium of growth and development that is core to this approach, and the belief that in each person, regardless of disability, ill health, disturbance or trauma, there is a part which can be reached through music and called into responsiveness, thereby enabling healing and the subsequent generalization into all aspects of a client's life. Nordoff and Robbins (1977) refer to this innate sensitivity to music as 'the Music Child', describing it as 'the individualized musicality inborn in each child: the term has reference to the universality of musical sensitivity – the heritage of complex sensitivity to the ordering and relationship of tonal and rhythmic movement; it also points to the distinctly personal significance of each child's musical responsiveness' (p.1).

My primary focus, therefore, is on the client's musical expression and on responding musically to the quality, timbre, pitch, dynamic, inflection and emotional feel of the client's speaking, crying, laughing, singing, instru- mental activity and body movements. However, as a therapist I feel that I have a responsibility to my clients to make all of myself and my experience available, as appropriate, to the therapy relationship and so I would also be flexible to travel where the client needs to go, using psychodynamic insights or words as appropriate and within my competence. My intent would then be to bring the work back into musical dialogue, with its rich diversity and potential to meet, reflect and intervene in order to bring about growth and change.

In the work with Danu, the child whom I write about in this chapter, the emphasis within the therapy process changed and developed, as you will see. At first, we worked solely within the music to find between us 'the ordering and relationship of tonal and rhythmic movement' described by Nordoff and Robbins (1977, p.1). As time went on we worked increasingly with issues from Danu's outside life, and here the 'distinctly personal significance' of Danu's musical being became more and more clear, as did her ability to use me as facilitator and fellow traveller on the therapeutic journey she devised.

Danu was a child with severe visual impairment, due to a rare brain disorder. She also had severe learning disabilities. However, during our work together in music therapy it soon became apparent that Danu's therapeutic needs lay in the area of what Sinason (1992) refers to as 'secondary handicap', rather than in her primary handicap of visual impairment. Sinason describes primary and secondary handicaps thus: 'In children or adults with an organic handicap, there is genetic, chromosomal or brain injury. This is real, measurable and incurable. However, the defensive use or abuse the individual makes of the primary damage can sometimes be more powerful than the original handicap itself' (p.112).

In Danu's case, her primary handicap was undoubtedly her visual impairment and brain disorder. The secondary handicaps which had initiated her referral to music therapy were depression, withdrawal and low cognitive functioning. Danu also smiled continuously, often inappropriately, and, on learning of her life circumstances, I was again reminded of Sinason, who writes of 'the handicapped smile' that so often is 'a defence against trauma' (p.136).

Danu was the child of Asian parents, whose marriage was arranged when Danu's mother was 15 years of age. Her mother resisted the marriage and was kept a virtual house prisoner until she reached her 16th birthday when she was sent overseas to meet and marry her husband. Danu was born 10 months later to a young, unhappy and angry mother who experienced great difficulty in accepting a disabled child. Bicknell (1981) writes of the grieving, mourning, anger, denial, rejection and guilt experienced by parents on the birth of a child with disability, even in a secure family base. How much more so, therefore, when family relationships are already under considerable strain, as was the case here.

Danu's background became one of emotional, physical and social deprivation and abuse. Her parents' marriage soon failed, resulting in separation when Danu was five years of age. For the next two years she lived sometimes with her father and sometimes with her mother, who, now having two younger children, found Danu's disability increasingly difficult. During this time, whilst living with her mother, school staff became increasingly worried about her health and Danu was placed on the child protection register because of evidence of bruising and because her parents had failed to give her essential health treatment for at least four months. She was found to be malnourished and dehydrated, suffering from acute starvation, with an untreated urinary-tract infection.

Because of the physical deprivation undergone whilst living with her mother, when Danu was seven her father was given custody of her. During this time she was constantly used as an emotional weapon between her parents, being allowed by her father to visit her mother at weekends when her parents were getting on relatively well but being refused visits at other times. When she did visit her mother's home, there were subsequent concerns, with Danu reporting that her mother hit and bruised her and the other children.

At this time Danu attended a school for children with visual impairment, where I was working as music therapist. When she was nine, the head teacher of the school referred her to me for music therapy. She described Danu as being so weak and physically frail that she could barely turn the hands of a play clock or chop a carrot in a cookery class. She had great difficulty concentrating and often fell asleep on the way to school in the bus, as well as during her lunch break and in class, and staff were understandably very concerned.

Early work

My first impression of Danu was of a physically small child, frail and underdeveloped, with extremely poor vision, unable to see more than a couple of inches in front of her and then only in a blurred and undefined way, who gingerly attempted the stairs leading down to the school music room. She presented as a very defended child, with an outwardly cheerful yet tense appearance, often giggling nervously. My aim at this point was to help her form a healthy and trusting relationship through the music and to help her connect with me in a less defended way.

In the initial sessions Danu played generally loudly and heavily with an erratic pulse, using all of the drums on the drum kit which was permanently set up in the large school music room. I supported this on piano, using strong diatonic chords and a variety of intervals, such as fourths, fifths and sevenths, while reflecting Danu's erratic pulse and rhythmic patterns. As she became aware of the piano meeting and reflecting her playing, so she began to dominate and test the relationship. It was hard to believe that this was the child who had been described to me as so frail and physically weak that she was hardly able to turn the hands of a play clock or chop a carrot.

There was considerable chaos in Danu's playing and her musical defences soon became very evident. This was illustrated in a variety of ways. To give one example, in a session three months into our work together, we were playing together in a 6/8 metre. Danu played loudly in quavers, initially accenting the first beat in each bar. She then began to either add or subtract a quaver from several bars, thus separating her accented beat from mine, potentially redefining the beginning of the bar. She also shifted from one instrument to another, changing rhythm and pulse again, moving away from musical connection. It was also noticeable how this apparently frail and physically weak child was able to play in a strong and controlling manner on the drum kit as I struggled musically to rejoin or even find a shared pulse.

Later in the same session Danu crouched down and reached up to play the instruments above her. Here, perhaps because of the sense of security and shieldedness of being hidden by the instruments, she seemed more able to allow the music to meet and connect with her rhythmically and, despite a few points where she momentarily moved away, this was the beginning of less resistance and more commitment to a shared two-way musical interaction.

Emergence of stories and songs

As the sessions continued, Danu began more and more to take a leading part in her own therapy and to use the sessions in many varying and dramatic ways, as will be seen. She was now more able to be involved in musical give-and-take exploration, responding to rhythmic phrases and using a large range of dynamics, tempi and timbre. She also began to use the entire room, dancing and using her voice expressively, apparently not limited by her poor vision. Whereas previously we had been working with the issues coming up within the musical relationship, we now also began to work more directly with outside issues and to move into the second stage of the therapy process. Here more and more questions arose for me – was it enough to be following her lead and journeying musically alongside her, playing supportive music for the exploration and expression of what I felt were deep, confusing and difficult emotions for this child? Alternatively, should I have been more directive, perhaps choosing a fairy story to encompass emerging witches and other characters, developing this into a personal story with uniquely devised songs and structures, as illustrated in some of the work of Nordoff and Robbins (1977)? The respective roles of words, music and psychodynamics was and is to the fore for me when thinking about this next phase with Danu. Was the therapy process in the words, in the music, in both, or in the psychodynamics of the relationship? When she was using her words dramatically, expressively, painfully or in song, was Danu inviting me to take heed of the words, the feelings or needs encompassed in the words and react and/or be proactive? Was she inviting or wishing me to interpret her words, make meaning of them and make them manageable, or did my musical support, acknowledgement and my listening address all of these aspects?

Four months into her therapy one of the older children in the school who travelled on the bus with Danu suddenly died, and all at the school were very upset. No one, however, had thought to tell me. But through the content of Danu's session that day I became aware of a change in her as she came into the session, and, for the first time, as she began to tell a story based on a children's book. With hindsight, I felt this was very much related to this boy's death.

> D: I'll tell you this story
> It's about a dark dark house
> Dark dark path
> And up the path was a dark dark house
> In the dark house was a dark dark staircase
> Up the dark dark stairs is a dark dark room
> In the dark dark room is a dark dark cupboard
> In the dark dark cupboard is a dark dark box
> In the dark dark box there was a –
> GHOST!

This was the beginning of weekly stories and dramatized songs. Generally, I could only pick up fragments of the words, partly due to the unsuitable acoustics in the room and also because Danu masked them by loud drum beats and cymbal crashes, as if not wanting them to be clearly heard at this stage. I therefore supported musically the intensity and mood of her stories as best I could, using the regularity of an ostinato bass to support sparse atonal music. During this period Danu would often crouch down behind the instruments, seeming to use them almost as a barrier between herself and me at the piano. Musically she was able to remain much more connected with me. I tended to play and sing atonally, wishing to allow her freedom of expression with no feeling of the expectation or demand which sometimes can be experienced when playing with a strongly defined tonal centre, and it seemed that this, along with the protective barrier of the drum kit, enabled her to risk being less musically defended.

Around this time Danu began to refer to the drum stick as 'stick' and her mother began to feature with phrases such as 'I'll tell my mother' and 'You'll tell my mother?…never.' She also began to use differentiated voices, one childlike and one harsh, and began to play the instruments in a punitive manner, as well as expressing considerable anger. This was illustrated by aggressive drum beating and her use of an angry kind of vocal recitative. Generally, I would support this with piano accompaniment, using an ostinato and dissonance within free improvisation to match the mood she was expressing as I usually could not hear her words. I felt that, as with using the instruments as a barrier, Danu was not yet quite ready to risk what a more direct expression – and connection – might bring.

In all this I felt strongly that at this point in the therapy Danu was acting out what she had experienced and seen.

Disclosure

As the sessions progressed Danu often sang about her mother, becoming increasingly clear in her vocal/verbal expression as she sang, asking why was her mother so bad; why had she left her? During this she often asked for certain music to be repeated to match specific moods or characters in her stories and songs, and I felt my role was to continue to support and facilitate her.

Over time, Danu gradually became more and more outgoing and assertive, both in and out of the therapy room. Eight months into her therapy she disclosed that she was being sexually abused by a friend of her father's. She made this disclosure to her mother, who refused to allow her to return to her father's house. I would like to illustrate how the music therapy process developed with words used in song by Danu in the ensuing sessions. The first four of these are from sessions after this disclosure when it was uncertain as to where she would continue to live, as her father still had legal custody of her.

The first excerpt is from a session one month after the disclosure. Earlier in the day Danu had said to her teacher: 'It was dark in my room, I was in my bed and I looked up and saw this funny thing. It looked as if it was wearing a coat with something on its head. It tried to get into bed with me. I saw it was my friend and I would not let him. When I looked again, he was in my sister's bed and she was on top of him. All the time my Auntie was snoring, snoring, snoring. I screamed out: "Mummy, Mummy, Mummy." Mummy came and said: "It's all right, Danu, it didn't happen. It was a dream."'

In her session later that day Danu sang/spoke the following in a strong assertive freely-pitched voice, whilst I accompanied her with sparsely-spaced, non-pulsed atonal chords:

> D: Am I dreaming, dreaming, dreaming, dreaming
> about sister?
> Am I dreaming, am I dreaming? No, I am *not*.
> Am I dreaming? No, I am *not* dreaming, no,
> Dreaming, dreaming, no-one is dreaming.

For a child who had suffered such trauma, it was an amazing example of her developing ego-strength that she could emphasize her belief in herself and her experience in this way.

This type of *'sprechgesang'* (speaking/singing) formed the major part of Danu's vocal expression in this phase of our work and was often best supported by spacious and free atonal music. I also felt that underpinning this with the regularity and predictability of ostinati or pedal notes helped to provide a containment for the painful feelings that Danu was expressing.

The next excerpt, from the same session, illustrates the pain and confusion that this child was feeling about where she belonged, having for most of her life been shunted between her parents, with her needs neglected and overlooked. Musically, I felt the need to move towards a more tonal experience to support this and contain these painful expressions but, as Danu constantly changed key throughout this poignant aria, it was almost impossible for me to be tonally together with her at this point.

> D: Today isn't a day for me. Where is everyone going?
> Home?
> No, not home.
> This is my home, this is where I live, this is where I want to

be.

No, no, no, no! This is not my home, this is – where is my real home?

Where is it? I want to see my real home, coming, coming, coming to me.

Where do I have a home? Where is it now?

I want to know. Where is my real home, where do I live?

Where is my home?

But most people know that 'there is my real home'. (therapist reflects)

Oh no, I don't know where my real home is – 'cause I know –

Where, tell me somebody, please tell me where my home is, where is my real home...

This was immediately followed by a cry for help and the music developed into a song with a strong rhythmic quality where the piano held and contained these very powerful emotions with clear harmonic structure and the use of major and minor thirds. Danu's emotional commitment to the expression of her inner dilemma and her emerging strength was reflected in her musical commitment and now we seemed tonally, rhythmically and expressively one with the music.

> D: Help me out, help me out, this can't be my home.
> Help me out, this can't be my real home.
> Won't somebody help me out, this can't be my home.
> Somebody help me out, this can't be my home.
> Somebody help me out, this can't be my real home.
> Somebody help me out, this can't be my real home.
> Help me out. Help me out. Help me out, somebody, somebody.
> Somebody help me out, help me somebody, help me out.
> Help me. Help me, help me out.
> Help me out now! Help me out now! Help me out now! Help me out now!

I noted earlier in this chapter that Danu had been diagnosed as having severe learning difficulties. My feeling had always been that her lack of cognitive ability and academic achievement was due to her emotional state and part of her secondary handicap. This is clearly illustrated in the next excerpt, from a session 20 months into her therapy. Here Danu was painfully poetic in her need for a home which she needed to be strong. The clarity of her words was noticeable and no longer needed to be masked by drum beats. I felt that she was now really able to trust that her message could, and should, be heard.

> D: I am your darkness. What do you call me?
> I will call you to make my home as good as anything, as good as gold.
> I may be the only one in this world to create this world.
> Who is there that is strong? Who can make my home good and strong? My home needs strongness. Please help me.
> I dare you, help me so that I – Oh look, some –
> I'll sing a song for you, or else I will play a tune for you. I –
> (harsh voice) I don't need you to have a house.
> (little voice) But sire, please, I need a home. I don't need anybody else's help, I only need yours.
> (harsh voice) What do you want from my home?
> (little voice) I really – (Danu curls up on the floor and whimpers)
> (harsh voice) Never mind.

Endings

Shortly after this Danu's mother regained legal custody. Some months later we had to finish music therapy, due both to the school closing and to Danu moving to another part of the country with her mother, brother and sister. In the interim period she was really able to consolidate her inner strength and develop a true sense of joy and fun in our music therapy together. Her dancing became creatively freer, supported by lively waltzes and energetic Middle Eastern-type music, and her singing became more song-like and melodic, indicating a real centring within herself, as well as containing a richness of expression and pleasure. That this consolidation has remained has been evident in the letters she sent me for the next two years, in which she told me about her new home and school.

My final excerpt is an example of how this amazing child dealt with our last session, where her strength was evident and her ability to handle the ending for both of us was so apparent in both her music, which was now tonal, rhythmic and clearly sung, and, as you will see here, in her words:

> D: (speaking, therapist supporting on piano) I was the only person that could not forget you. Because this time it's not gonna be memories. You've got your mind still with me

inside it. So, don't be upset, just say to yourself – Oh no, she's not gone, she's still left in your mind, and you'll never forget it. So, don't howl about it...

Th: (singing) 'Cause you'll still be in my mind,

D: (singing) Oh no, there'll still be memories,

Th: We'll still be in our minds,

D: I'll be still there!

Th: So we'll always remember each other.

D: I'll still be there.

D: (speaking again) So don't forget, you'll be in my mind, and I'll be in yours, so we both won't forget each other. And we won't forget to write to each other, and don't forget, because I'll give you my address, so you can write to me back.

Th: (singing) I'll write to you, and you'll write to me, so we'll be in each other's minds.

Th/D: (singing) We'll remember, we'll remember, we'll remember the stories and songs we sang; we'll remember, we'll remember each other, memories – (Danu beats the drums)

D: (speaking) But now this is the only time I'll be playing on these drums, so... (she plays strongly again)

Conclusion

The process that Danu and I shared posed many clinical questions for me, the answers to some of which remain unresolved. However, what seems without doubt is that music therapy was vitally important for Danu. It allowed her to be musically 'in control', something which patently had been altogether removed from her life. In the music she could dominate and test the security of our musical relationship by rejecting and resisting it, and find freedom of expression. My musical support, acceptance and facilitating of her through the music enabled her to discover that our musical relationship was strong enough and flexible enough to hold, contain and support the experiencing and expression of traumatically painful feelings. It also freed her creativity, thereby helping her rediscover her inner strength and sense of self, and enabled her to become a creative, energetic and joyful 12-year-old.

Glossary

Ego-strength: a sense of self and of one's central personality as being sound and strong.

Music child: 'That entity in every child that responds to musical experience.' (Nordoff and Robbins 1977, p.1)

Musical defences: musical 'habits' or unconscious ways of playing which are used to avoid or move away from musical connection within the relationship with the therapist.

Ostinato: a pattern of notes that is repeated over and over again.

Reflecting: providing a musical portrait of the client's responses.

Sprechgesang: vocal speech/song of the 20th century avant-garde musical school.

Strongly defined tonal centre: a pull towards the first note or tonal centre of a scale.

References

Bicknell, D.J. (1981) *Living with a Mentally Handicapped Member of the Family.* London: St George's Medical School Hospital.

Nordoff, P. and Robbins, C. (1971) *Therapy in Music for Handicapped Children.* London: Gollancz.

Nordoff, P. and Robbins, C. (1977) *Creative Music Therapy.* New York: John Day Company.

Sinason, V. (1992) *Mental Handicap & The Human Condition.* London: Free Association Books.

CHAPTER 9

Orff Music Therapy with Multi-Handicapped Children
Melanie Voigt

Introduction

Developmental disabilities are complex phenomena. They often affect more than one area of development, resulting in 'multiple handicaps'. A child with a cerebral motor disability, such as cerebral palsy, may have great difficulty in moving at all, resulting in a lack of incentive to use his motor abilities to explore surroundings. This lack of stimulation can prevent him from having experiences necessary for positive social and emotional development and for the development of perceptual abilities. A child with learning disabilities may have trouble understanding specific situations, making it difficult to cope with changes in the environment. This can lead to states of anxiety or to the development of stereotyped behaviours. The child who is affected by a visual impairment receives less information from his environment and can have trouble in orientation within a room. Social signals from others may not be perceived.

A developmental disability not only affects the child and his development, it also plays a role in the development of relationships between the child and his family and the relationship of the other family members to another as well (Sarimski 1993; Turnbull *et al.* 1986). Therapeutic approaches used to treat children with these problems must be adapted to the developmental profile of the patient and consider his family situation and social environment.

Clinical background

The goals of social paediatrics are the early diagnosis and therapy of developmental disabilities and the integration of developmentally disturbed children within the family and society. Gertrud Orff developed an approach to music therapy within this setting specifically for treatment of children with developmental problems and disabilities. Orff Music Therapy is an integral part of the interdisciplinary concept of the *Kinderzentrum München*, the first centre for social pediatrics in Munich, Germany.

A large number of patients treated at the *Kinderzentrum München* are children and youths who have multiple handicaps. Often, these children must be led to develop an interest in events, objects and persons in their environments. They must be offered the opportunity to interact at their personal levels of competency while being supported in developing these further. Many of these children receive treatment in the music therapy department. Music therapy offers them the opportunity to experience the successful effects of their own activities, to express themselves at their individual developmental levels and to develop new possibilities of interaction and communication. Parents often need support and suggestions for play as well as the opportunity to experience their children in a positive way. They can be involved in the music therapy setting actively or passively and can receive support and suggestions for positive interaction with their children.

Orff Music Therapy

The elements of Orff Music Therapy are sound and movement, which work together in a stimulating situation of play. The combination of these phenomena – play and an acoustical atmosphere – is viewed as being helpful in providing the child with the opportunity for experiencing, testing and confirming self-affirmation, understanding for others and social integration (Orff 1980). The importance of play for positive development is supported by research in the area of developmental psychology and is also considered important for the development of a positive parent–child relationship and for the quality of emotional attachment (Hughes 1995; Rubin, Fein and Vandenberg 1983). Musical activities within a play situation can provide a possibility for self-expression and for the development of social and interactive competencies.

Characteristics of therapy

Orff Music Therapy is an *active* form of music therapy. All patients, including those with severe multiple handicaps, are involved in musical activities. The different developmental processes and abilities of the children determine the types of activities employed.

Orff Music Therapy is *child centered*. The basic attitude towards the patients is similar to that found in humanistic psychology (Bruscia 1987; Vocke 1986). Patients with developmental disabilities are seen as having potential for positive development and self-actualization within the framework of their handicaps or disability. Although Orff Music Therapy was not developed with a particular theory of psychotherapy in mind, the attitude described above represents a principle of client-centered therapy (Bruscia 1987; Smeijsters 1994; Vocke 1986). This attitude, supplemented with knowledge of human development, particularly developmental psychology, forms the basis for therapeutic procedures. As in psychotherapy, Orff Music Therapy takes place within a state of encounter between therapist and patient, making the relationship between them a central factor in the therapy (Orff 1980). The therapist acts as a mediator for the child's development, motivating and supporting the development of his strengths and personality (Orff 1980, 1989). In order to achieve this goal, she must be open, accepting, genuine and empathetic. At the same time, she needs to be consequent, to be clear in her behaviour, to be able to observe herself and the child and to know and recognize the possibilities and limitations of the child as well as her own limitations. She must have authority without being authoritarian (Orff 1989).

Orff Music Therapy is defined as *developmental music therapy* (Bruscia 1989). It takes into account not only cognitive, motor, auditory or visual development but social and emotional development and, hence, personality development as well. The patient's family background, his personal history and development, his feelings and his personality development are regarded and the therapeutic measures taken are adapted to meet the needs of each individual patient (Bruscia 1989). This requires that the therapist have knowledge of the various developmental processes affecting the child so that his needs can be met adequately.

Method of application

In Orff Music Therapy it is assumed that the child will be able to act and interact with the therapist. This is considered possible if the therapist accepts the child as he is and approaches the child in a way that reflects his personality and development. Gertrud Orff uses the word 'ISO', meaning the same or similar, to describe this behaviour of the therapist. The word 'provocation' is used to describe the behaviour of the therapist in which she introduces new stimuli or impulses with the intention of helping the child broaden his ability to act (Orff 1980, 1989). Observation of the child's behaviour – for example, his interests and initiative, his strengths and weaknesses, his reactions to sounds, activities or impulses brought into the situation by the adult – form the basis for the activities of the therapist and for the evaluation of therapy. The behaviour of the child is viewed within the total context of his development, not as an isolated event in itself.

These principles correspond to the principles of responsive interaction which combine humanistic ideals and developmental psychology. It is assumed that the child will show interests and initiative for activity and/or interaction. This assumption implies that a potential to act is existent. The therapist observes the behaviour of the child and is willing to accept ideas and initiative from him and to enter into interaction with him at these levels (Sarimski 1993).

The principles of responsive interaction also allow for the fact that the child can, or will, encounter difficulties in acting or interacting and that it can be necessary for help to be given from an outside source – in this case the therapist. The therapist then adapts her support to the developing competence of the child. The form of help given should involve the child actively in the process of acquiring new ways of acting and/or interacting positively with her environment so that these new competencies can be internalized and development can take place (Sarimski 1993). Responsive interaction seems to show a positive effect in areas such as concentration, dealing with challenging situations independently and the development of the parent–child–relationship (Hughes 1995; Sarimski 1993).

These principles allow the therapist to be flexible in interacting with the child in such a way that his/her personal needs can be met. Used together with active music making within a situation of play, they form the basis on which the therapeutic process in Orff Music Therapy takes place. The child is not pressed into a specific therapy 'programme' but the therapy is adapted flexibly to meet the needs which are a result of his/her individual developmental processes.

Descriptions of musical material

The musical material used in Orff Music Therapy is influenced by four factors: music understood in the sense of *musiké*, improvisation, the instruments used and the multi-sensory aspects of music.

MUSIC

In Orff Music Therapy music is understood in the sense of *musiké*, meaning 'a total presentation in word, sound and movement' (Orff 1980, p.9). Instruments, non-musical objects and body instruments can produce sound. Vocalization, as well as complex verbalization, comprise the content of speech, which can be rhythmic or meditative. Movement in music therapy can range from a facial expression or a spontaneous motion of a part of the body to movement as dance and to inner movement (feelings – for example, to be moved by something) (Orff 1980, 1989). This broad definition of music differs from that usually used today in which music is considered to be a 'complex of organized sounds' (Orff 1980, p.9). It can include activities such as 'playing with sound', melodic and rhythmic performance or role-play and enables us to develop a wide variety of activities in which the developmentally disabled child can be an active participant.

IMPROVISATION

The idea of creative, spontaneous music making is central in Orff Music Therapy. Its purpose is to provide a creative stimulus for the child (Orff 1980). This does not mean that one only plays 'freely'. Structure or form is present through the music itself – for example, playing/not playing; sound/silence (Orff 1989). Improvisation also includes spontaneous play. For Orff, musical activity and play both include the ordered and predetermined, and the unordered and undetermined (Orff 1980). In musical play the player's partner can be an instrument or another person, depending on whether he plays alone or with someone else (Orff 1989). One can investigate materials, build complexes of sound or build in the literal sense, practice through play – exploring different possibilities of making music – and associate sounds with ideas, moods or situations when playing with music (Orff 1989).

INSTRUMENTS

In Orff Music Therapy the traditional Orff instruments are used together with instruments such as the lyre, piano, monochord and various percussion instruments, as well as electronic keyboards. This wide variety of instruments provides many possibilities for producing musical sounds, even for the severely handicapped.

The instruments themselves allow and encourage active participation. They provide a link between therapist and child, enable both closeness and distance and provide a means of communicating and practising social skills. Orff considers the communicative possibilities of the instruments to be three-fold: between child and material, between child and therapist via the material, between two children (Orff 1980).

In addition to musical instruments, non-musical materials such as scarves, balls, marbles, a marble tower, hand puppets, chains of beads, chalk boards, etc. are used in the play situation to allow the child a wide variety of possibilities to express himself within the idea of musiké. The musical instruments and the non-musical play materials also provide multi-sensory aspects which can be included in the musical play situation.

MULTI-SENSORY ASPECTS OF MUSIC

The multi-sensory aspects of music are implicit in the idea of musiké. They are included in the therapeutic process and can aid the therapist in meeting the needs and furthering the development of the patients (Bruscia 1989; Orff 1980). According to Orff, the multi-sensory aspects of music can '1. heighten perceptive awareness, 2. encourage associative thinking, 3. compensate for a deficiency in one of the senses, 4. develop more economical musical ideas' (Orff 1989, p.26). Multi-sensory activities serve to help integrate different modalities. They serve to motivate a child who is yet unable or unwilling to participate in musical activities to enter into interaction and, with time, to accept musical interaction. Children feel the sound of a drum through its vibrations. This sensation can be used to catch their attention, to cause relaxation or stimulation, or to provide them with a feeling in parts of the body which they do not normally use. The multi-sensory aspects of active music making can support cognitive processes through the integration of different basic skills in the areas of auditory, visual, motor, language and social development (Nocera 1979). Being able to perform a musical activity, to order the elements used and to carry out motor, auditory, visual, language and social tasks, can challenge the child's mental and social potentials. For example, children must be able to integrate the basic skills mentioned above and, additionally, show adequate social competencies in order for a musical activity to be carried out to the satisfaction of all those involved.

Developing musical material

Musical material can be developed by using a traditional rhyme, verse or song as a basic idea for the development of an activity within the situation at hand; improvising on a word, sound, motion or musical fragment which the child expresses spontaneously within the therapy setting; playing instruments freely within a given structure, such as question and answer or solo and tutti form; combining musical elements with role-play, drawing or multi-sensory elements using musical instruments and non-musical materials. Some musical materials can be planned before therapy, some worked out within the therapy session and others occur when situations in therapy lead to improvisation. Important in the development of musical material is the idea of economy. 'Our maxim is to make a little go a long way' (Orff 1989, p.73). A limited amount of material is not considered restrictive, it provides a basis from which abundance can develop.

The therapist plays with the child using musical means, always with the principles of development in mind. By observing the child's behaviour, she can 'determine which musical stimuli would be appropriate; also how and to what extent they should be used' (Orff 1989, pp.11–12). For example, she can act musically to support or develop an acoustical atmosphere which corresponds to or sets the mood of the situation. The improvisation of 'situation songs' – songs which arise out of a specific situation – can enable her to give signals, to structure, to comment or mirror, to react. The introduction of new musical elements or structures can gain the attention of the child and/or motivate him to new activity.

This role requires adequate musical competencies of the therapist. The therapist using Orff Music Therapy must understand music and possess musical skills to the extent that she can react spontaneously and competently within the therapy situation. A thorough knowledge of the elements of music and the ability to use these to meet the child at his level of development are necessary in order to develop musical materials which are appropriate.

Clinical example

Sandra, a girl with severe learning disabilities, is two years and nine months old at the beginning of music therapy. The exact cause of her disability is not clear. The possibility of a metabolic or genetic disorder has not been excluded. Developmental assessment shows that she demonstrates cognitive abilities corresponding to those of an eight-month-old child. Her gross motor abilities appear to be unsteady. Expressive language is not present, the extent of language comprehension is not clear. She does almost nothing with her hands, with the exception of carrying out stereotyped motions. The family finds it difficult to discover activities which interest her, things she wants to do or seems to enjoy. Sandra is referred to music therapy with the following goal: development of possibilities for communicative behaviour.

Session 1

The goal of the first session with Sandra was to establish contact and possibilities for interaction with her and to observe her behaviour in order to determine where her strengths and weaknesses lay. I sang a short song in greeting, she listened, making eye contact. Sandra stood, looked at her mother who sat at the edge of the room, looked around the room, apparently trying to orient herself to the new surroundings but exploring nothing. She put her left hand repeatedly in her mouth and held the right, formed to a fist, in the air, moving it at the wrist and kneading her fingers.

Clearly structured musical material was used to intensify contact and begin interaction. I played a lively rhythm on the drum, eight measures in 2/4 time, which I exactly repeated once. She looked over to me, seeming to show interest. She began walking around the room without clearly approaching anyone or anything. The rhythm described above formed the basic accompaniment for rhythmic speech and a situation song, the text of which commented on our activities – my playing the drum, her movement within the room ('dancing'). Pauses were made at the completion of each repetition. In these pauses Sandra again looked at me, smiled, stood still. She directed her attention towards my activity and engaged in eye contact. Her facial expression conveyed a positive reaction to my activity.

Using the principle of provocation, I played a drum roll with my fingers. Sandra came to the drum spontaneously and put her hands on the drumhead. I repeated the drum roll with my fingers. She experienced the sound in a multi-sensory way, hearing it and feeling the vibrations simultaneously. She looked at me wide-eyed. As she lifted her hands, I ceased to produce sound. She went away but could be motivated to return through a repetition of the drum roll, and again she placed her hands on the drum. She wandered around the drum, looking interested but not becoming actively involved. As I placed my arm lightly across her back in order to make clear where the activity was taking place, it seemed she received the orientation she needed. At this point she placed her fingers on the drum repeatedly, letting the drum roll 'tickle' them. In the pauses she made intensive eye contact. Shortly thereafter, Sandra hit the drum with her hand one time. I answered with one beat on the drum and reinforced her activity socially, then repeated the situation song from the beginning of the session, commenting on her activity. This sequence took place three times before Sandra's interest waned and she moved away from the drum. During this second set of activities she had entered into contact with an object, accepted the requirement that she remain at the drum and began to show signs of playing in a dialogue-like way as well as making social contact and conveying her reactions to what was taking place.

At this point, 25 minutes had passed. Because of her developmental problems, Sandra needed time to orient herself within the new situation, to get to know and accept a person who was a stranger to her, and to arrive at the point at which she was able to participate musically in an active way. Sandra's motor problems made it difficult for her to sit alone and do something with her hands at the same time. She also appeared to have difficulty at times in understanding and carrying out the activities. Subsequent activities (playing the lyre, playing a simple circle game) seemed too difficult or too demanding. She refused to participate, beginning to cry. This behaviour conveyed her feelings and her difficulties, causing me to revise my own behaviour – to accept her negative reaction and to observe her behaviour again for signs of interest or preference.

She went to a shelf, looking at the objects on it without touching any of them or showing a clear preference in an observable way. I took a string of gold-coloured beads and offered Sandra the opportunity to get to know them by using multi-sensory aspects of the material. I moved the beads over her wrists, letting them lightly touch the skin, chanting, in a rocking rhythm, 'Back and forth, and back and forth, and back and forth and still.' Somewhat later the beads were raised above her head and shaken, making a rustling sound. When I sang 'Where are the beads?' on a minor third, as if a peek-a-boo game was being played, she reacted by looking up at the beads!

During this ten-minute activity Sandra began to make contact with the beads herself. She shook them and actively sought them when they were out of sight but could still be heard. The session was brought to a close with a farewell song which was used in all subsequent sessions. She had again accepted my suggestion for activity, had made contact with the material involved and began to explore it. She took part in a mutual game at her developmental level.

During this first session Sandra exhibited the ability to make social contact with persons through eye contact. She expressed positive and negative reactions to activities, music and objects but did not vary her behaviour to make concrete wishes known. She was willing to accept suggestions and requirements that I initiated but took no initiative herself. The activities used needed to be very simple, corresponding to her cognitive abilities. Her movement within the room seemed aimless and the stereotyped movements of her hands made it difficult for her to use them to explore objects or cause effects.

Course of therapy

Sandra's seemingly aimless movement around the room provided an opportunity to use traditional circle games or to develop movement games in which a distinct musical structure determined movement and rest. This contrast between walking and standing, corresponding to sound and silence, made it possible to catch Sandra's attention repeatedly. At the same time, she was experiencing structure within interaction. Her mother was included in the games and supported Sandra when necessary. Her favourite game seemed to be one in which the drum accompanied the song. Her mien during the pauses preceding the repetition of the song suggested that she anticipated the next round. She especially seemed to look forward to the 'songless' parts of the game, for when she heard the words 'On your mark, get set, go!' she looked at me and laughed joyfully. Sandra was now taking part in mutual musical games, following the sequence, carrying out the activity and responding to signals within a given structure.

The fact that Sandra did not take the initiative or try to make herself understood by varying her behaviour made it difficult for her family to know what interested her or what she wanted to do. In therapy she began to show tendencies towards initiative by approaching different instruments in the room. These signs of initiative provided a possibility for developing mutual activities. When she approached an instrument, we either played it together or took turns. This supported her interest in her surroundings and helped her develop the ability to communicate her wishes in some way. She soon began to show preferences, especially for keyboard instruments. If I did not understand her or did not react to her behaviour, she returned to the instrument repeatedly until I lifted her onto the stool. At first, Sandra played mostly with her left hand, producing clusters on the keyboard. She played these usually only once and for a relatively short time. I answered in the pauses in a similar way but with variations in frequency and tempo. Occasionally, she played spontaneously with her right hand, which was normally held in the air and moved in a stereotyped way. Through these activities we developed a way of playing together musically which more and more began to resemble a dialogue. Sandra looked at me when she was through playing and waited until I had finished my part before beginning to play again. Sandra had begun to show initiative and to vary her behaviour so that she could make her wishes known. She was able to take turns, a skill necessary for communication and dialogue.

The difficulties she had in using her hands to carry out activities was another factor which hindered her ability to interact with objects and to experience different possibilities of acting. Her first contact with instruments – drum, piano, stringed instruments – occurred with the hand directly. Other instruments required a 'tool' – for example, a mallet – in order for a satisfying sound to be produced. At the beginning of therapy Sandra did not understand this principle. The mallet usually found its way to her mouth and the instrument remained silent. The opportunity to take part in activities requiring this ability was offered repeatedly. Only enough support was given to enable her to carry out the activity herself. For example, I supported her arm lightly at the elbow so that her spontaneous wrist movements would cause the mallet to hit the instrument and produce sound. The first musical sounds were produced by chance, then with increasing intention until no more support was needed. Sandra's stereotyped activities with her hands seemed be a symptom of a problem of planning actions, not of avoiding contact, since she showed no aversion when touching or being touched. Through the activities described above, it was possible to observe an increase in her ability to carry out activities using her hands intentionally.

Session 17

At the end of the well-known and well-liked movement game described above, Sandra was asked, through a situation song, where she would like to play next. She went straight over to the piano! At first, she played with both hands, then mainly with the left. Her music consisted of clusters with an occasional single tone, usually played with her forefinger on a black key. She varied her position on the keys between middle C and the F below it, playing sequences of up to eleven tones pre-rhythmically with a feeling of quarters and eighths, punctuated by notes held slightly longer or by short pauses. She played alone and in dialogue with me. At times we played together, her playing directing mine. She often made eye contact with me between musical episodes, smiling. Later on in the session she played the cymbal without help, using a mallet. She played pre-melodic sequences of five notes in a feeling of eighths on the pentatonic pipe glockenspiel, pausing after the fifth note. This made it possible to answer her in a similar way, again creating a musical dialogue.

Observations made after these seventeen sessions in therapy showed that Sandra was using her gross and fine motor skills intentionally to achieve certain effects and attain certain goals. In the areas of interaction, communication and social competence we observed that she initiated activities and interaction and modified her behaviour in order to make her wishes understood. This made it possible for her to influence events. Her musical behaviour had changed immensely since the beginning of therapy. She now played pre-rhythmic and pre-melodic sequences, using her hands in different ways or using a 'tool', creating differences in sound.

Relationship of theory to practice

The course of music therapy with Sandra, described above, illustrates the elements, characteristics and method of Orff Music Therapy. Sandra was actively involved in the therapy setting. Activities and goals were geared to her developmental competencies and needs. The desire to be able to involve Sandra more in daily activities and to be able to understand her wishes were needs expressed by her family. These were also taken into account. Sandra showed strength in the area of social interest. This strength was supported in therapy using activities in which direct interaction between persons played an important part. The problems she had in planning her own actions, caused by the cognitive disability, resulted in difficulty carrying out activities. Here she was offered support until she was able to successfully carry out the activity herself – for example, playing with a mallet or making her wishes known. Multi-sensory aspects of music were used to provide information for Sandra through more than one modality. Feeling the vibrations of an instrument and combining movement and sound are two examples here. The instruments and musical activities motivated her to make more contact with objects in her environment and to come to terms with them actively. Through this active involvement with objects and persons in her environment she developed new interests and means of communicating these.

My role as therapist was to discover and support her strengths and to provide musical activities within a setting of responsive interaction in order to promote development. It was necessary that I understand her developmental problems and processes and, at the same time, be willing to see that she also had strengths on the basis of which we could interact. I needed to meet her at her own level, not at the level at which I would have liked her to be. This meant that I needed to respond to her music in a similar way when we were playing together – for example, by answering pre-melodically and pre-rhythmically instead of playing a clearly structured melody. At the same time, I needed to provide her with a stimulating situation. Here the ability to improvise melodically and rhythmically was necessary in order to develop situation songs and movement activities which would generate excitement and interest. When she had difficulty, I gave her just enough help to enable her to use the abilities she had in experiencing new possibilities of acting and interacting. The observation of Sandra's behaviour made it possible to act and react adequately, as well as to determine her developmental progress.

Role of observation

Orff stresses the importance of the observation of the child's behaviour as the basis for planning and carrying out therapy (Orff 1980, 1989). The first step in this process is the *establishment of indications and goals* for therapy. The traditional categories of the different developmental disabilities only serve as a point of orientation for working with handicapped children in music therapy. The developmental problems described are not always characteristic of a single form of developmental disability. We often find overlapping characteristics which are influenced through the individual developmental processes of the child. For this reason, we do not use only the diagnosis as a point of reference to determine the indication to therapy but observe the individual characteristics of the child's development and behaviour as well. It is the duty of the therapist to define the indication and goals precisely on the basis of her observations within the therapy setting.

In Sandra's case it was not the learning disability alone which determined the indication to therapy. Rather, the problems she had resulting from the learning disability – making contact with her environment and interacting with persons and objects – formed the indication for therapy. The goals pursued began with focusing her attention and motivating her to make contact with persons and objects through the medium of music. As these goals were reached, new goals – such as the development of the ability to follow a sequence of play, the support of initiative and communicative behaviours, the development of musical dialogue and the development of new skills for carrying out activities – were formulated and pursued.

Observation of behaviour is also used in the *evaluation of progress* in therapy. In Orff Music Therapy we do not interpret behaviour without looking at the child's broader, developmental context. We use principles of observation in which the behaviours to be observed and the goal of the interaction being observed are clearly defined. Activities, events and behaviours are described concretely within the context of the interaction taking place. Interpretations of, or speculations about, behaviour are avoided or identified as such. The use of clearly defined items within the categories of interaction and communication, social behaviour, motor skills and musical behaviour enabled me to describe Sandra's progress in therapy and to note what was changing in her development.

The emphasis on the observation of behaviour does not exclude the possibility that developmental processes take place covertly within the area of feeling and emotion. On the contrary, 'inner movement' or emotion is considered to be vital to the processes of development and therapy (Orff 1989). Changes in interaction, observed within the therapy setting, can give us clues about the social and emotional development of the child.

Possible benefits of Orff Music Therapy

In our clinical experience the use of musical activities and materials within a developmental and responsive approach to therapy often provides a 'breakthrough' in fundamental areas of development. Major areas of our work include therapy with children having the following developmental disabilities and problems: multiple handicaps, cerebral palsy, hearing impairments, autism, behaviour disorders, learning disabilities and language disorders.

Another area of benefit that we have been able to observe is in the area of parental involvement. Parenting style is known to have an important influence on social and emotional development (Durkin 1995). Rubin, Fein and Vandenberg (1983) suggest that the social and emotional aspects of play are possibly as important for the adult (e.g. parents) as they are for the child.

Parents of children with developmental disabilities frequently feel helpless and uncertain because, often, their children are not able to respond as expected to their suggestions for play and interaction. Uncertainty in setting boundaries, in challenging the child without demanding too much of him and in playing with him can provide the basis for problems in parent-child interaction. These problems, in turn, can represent a secondary risk to the child's development (Sarimski 1993). The parents' experience in the therapy process can enable them to incorporate principles observed and discussed in music therapy within play situations in everyday life. Sandra's mother took part in therapy, both as an observer and as an active participant. She used principles she had observed and experienced in therapy in playing with her child. Musical instruments that the family possessed played an important part in interaction with Sandra.

Summary

Orff Music Therapy is a developmental approach to music therapy. The child is considered to have a creative potential within the framework of his developmental problems. Music, understood in the sense of *musiké*, is employed in a situation of play using principles of responsive interaction to support and further the patients in different areas of development. These principles reflect the mixture of humanistic ideals and developmental psychology mirrored in the procedures of Orff Music Therapy. Music, in the broad sense of the word *musiké*, makes it possible to involve a wide spectrum of children with developmental disabilities and problems actively in the therapeutic process and to help them realize their developmental potentials.

Glossary

Developmental music therapy: music therapy that is used to treat patients of any age who are experiencing disturbances in any area of developmental processes. It may be concerned with specific medical or physical problems as well as with personality development and personal feelings. The procedures used are adapted to meet the needs of the patients (Bruscia 1989).

ISO: the same, similar. The therapist encounters the child in a way that is in accord with the interests and nature of the child (Orff 1980, 1989).

Pre-melodic: '…"musical" expression which results in no recognizable melody (in the accepted sense) and cannot be repeated … Physical impulses working on a melodic playing surface produce a pre-melodic style' (Orff 1989, p.46).

Pre-rhythmic: '…usually coupled with pre-melodic playing – a free rhythmic flow with no fixed structure or regular pulse (barring)' (Orff 1989, p.43).

Provocation: new stimuli and impulses introduced by the therapist with the intention of helping the child to broaden his abilities to act and interact (Orff 1980, 1989).

Responsive interaction: an approach to interaction in which the adult is willing to accept ideas and initiatives of the child and to enter into interaction with the child at these levels. He adapts his support to the developing competence of the child, involving the child actively in overcoming difficulties and developing new possibilities of behaviour and interaction (Sarimski 1993).

Social paediatrics: a branch of paediatrics in Germany. Its basic goal is the early diagnosis and early therapy of developmental disorders within an interdisciplinary setting.

References

Bruscia, K. (1987) *Improvisational Models of Music Therapy.* Springfield: Charles C. Thomas Publishers.

Bruscia, K. (1989) *Defining Music Therapy.* Phoenixville: Barcelona Publishers.

Durkin, K. (1995) *Developmental Social Psychology from Infancy to Old Age.* Oxford: Blackwell Publishers.

Hughes, F.P. (1995) *Children, Play & Development* (2nd Edition). Boston: Allyn and Bacon.

Nocera, S.D. (1979) *Reaching the Special Learner through Music.* Morristown: Silver Burdett.

Orff, G. (1980) *The Orff Music Therapy.* Translated by Margaret Murray. New York: Schott Music Corporation.

Orff, G. (1989) *Key Concepts in the Orff Music Therapy.* Translated by Jeremy Day and Shirley Salmon. London: Schott Music Corporation.

Rubin, K.H., Fein, G.C. and Vandenberg, B. (1983) 'Play.' In E.M. Hetherington (ed.) *Handbook of Child Psychology. Vol.4: Socialization, Personality and Social Development.* New York: Wiley.

Sarimski, K. (1993) *Interaktive Frühförderung.* Weinheim: Psychologie-Verlags-Union.

Smeijsters, H. (1994) *Musiktherapie als Psychotherapie. Grundlagen, Ansätze, Methoden.* Stuttgart: Fischer.

Turnbull, A.P., Turnbull, H.R., Summers, J.A., Brotherson, M.J. and Benson, H.A. (1986) *Families and Professionals: Creating an Exceptional Partnership.* Columbus: Merrill Publishing Co.

Vocke, J. (1986) *Effektivitätskontrolle der Orff-Musiktherapie.* Dissertation. Munich: Ludwig-Maximilians-Universität.

CHAPTER 10

The Music, the Meaning, and the
Therapist's Dilemma

Sandra Brown

Introduction

When I began work with Peter, he was ten-and-a-half years old. He was diagnosed as being at the 'high-functioning' end of the autistic spectrum but was incapable, in many ways, of dealing with his world, cognitively, socially and emotionally. He spoke in a monotone voice, had many obsessive behaviours and was very isolated, with no real contact or relationships within his peer group or with staff at school. Peter was referred to music therapy because of the staff's concerns over his apparent negative self-image. He wouldn't look at himself in the mirror and he refused to listen to his name, calling himself by other names. He also talked frequently of killing himself and there were very real fears for his safety.

Wing (1993) describes the person with autism as having a 'triad of social impairments', with difficulties arising in reciprocal social relationships, in communication, both verbal and non-verbal, and in the development of play and imagination. Stereotypic and obsessive behaviours are also typical in people with autism, which may result from efforts to deal with the 'confusing interacting mass of events, places, sounds and sights' (Jollife, Lansdown and Robinson 1992, p.14) which is the reality of life for many autistic people.

The severity of these difficulties varies across a broad spectrum, from the severely communicatively disabled child or adult with no speech and little connection with the world outside, to the child like Peter, who, in some areas, could appear quite competent, but whose understanding and interaction in many other areas was quite severely impaired.[1]

Peter and I worked together for four-and-a-half years in once-weekly individual music therapy sessions, each lasting for half an hour. Throughout that time what was going on in my head in terms of clinical thought changed, both according to the material that Peter brought and in relation to the progression of the therapy itself. The questions which arose for me from this in some ways reflect the dilemma of many music therapists working in the UK, where there is a continuum – and, sometimes, polarity – of views concerning the essential nature of music therapy. These views vary widely, from the psychotherapeutic to the phenomenological, as can be seen in John (1992) writing that 'music is a useful link in the chain of processes from the unconscious…to consciousness and its attendant words' (p.12) and Ansdell (1995) writing that 'the heart of the therapy is contained within the music – an experience which is allowed to speak for itself' (p.32).

As a music therapist trained in the Nordoff–Robbins tradition (see Nordoff and Robbins 1971, 1977), a belief in the musical process itself as an instrument of change in its own right is central to my work, and, in the work with Peter, the heart of the therapy was indeed contained within the music, as you will see. However, as we progressed I drew on other models in thinking about the work, both developmentally and in consideration of the psychological and symbolic nature of some of Peter's material, as well as my awareness of countertransferential feelings and images, particularly at one point in the work. The dilemma then arose for me: were these extra-musical considerations unnecessary, self-indulgent, even clouding the music therapy work? Was listening and responding clinically within the musical clinical model, as indeed I was, an effective therapeutic process in itself, where the work was happily taking place without these extraneous thoughts, which served only as an intellectual interest for me? The result of these explorations will be seen in the following pages and will, I hope, serve to stimulate your own thoughts on the matter.

1   Much has been written about the value of music therapy for people with autism and, for the sake of brevity, I would refer interested readers to Brown (1994) and Trevarthen *et al.* (1996) for more detailed views of current research in the field.

Exposition

When Peter and I began working together his instrumental playing was turbulent and erratic, often without pulse or any relationship to what I might play. The therapy room contained a variety of tuned and untuned percussion instruments, as well as a piano, and Peter consistently played a very resonant drum and a cymbal, with occasional playing of the piano. In his drum and cymbal playing his physical movements were exaggerated and compulsive, and he seemed absorbed in what Nordoff and Robbins (1971) called 'emotional-force beating' – 'engrossed in fulfilling his emotional and muscular impulses in the amount of noise he can generate' without any 'stable or constructive rhythmic responses' (p.67). Here my aim, through creative improvisation, was to match and reflect the qualities of Peter's playing in order to give him an externalized experience of himself in relation to me, while trying to develop points of awareness and shared musical meaning.

This first period of work was, therefore, informed by a creative musical therapeutic model (see Figure 10.1). My aims here were to do with forming a musical relationship, meeting and reflecting Peter's playing, enabling him to listen, working for the development of musical components such as pulse, rhythm, dynamic, etc. I also had more general therapeutic aims, such as building a working therapeutic relationship and providing and holding a

1	Musical	a)	working through clinical musical techniques; musical analysis and aims
		b)	creating a musical–emotional environment
2	Developmental (with consideration of pathology)		e.g. autism – possible deficits in:
		a)	communication skills (turn taking, listening skills, etc.)
		b)	play and imagination
		c)	difficulty in understanding/relating to own/others' emotions (cf. Wing 1993)
3	Psychodynamic		e.g. concepts of: frame, regression, early psychological development (cf. Klein, Winnicott, Stern), countertransference, containment (cf. Bion)

Figure 10.1 Models

containing frame for the therapy process, but my mind's eye – and ear – was on musical elements.

Throughout the following months Peter continued to play with enormous volume, and with no apparent recognition of me as an 'active music person' in relation to him (cf. Nordoff and Robbins 1977, p.184). Any attempts I made to encourage alternative modes of playing together – for example, introducing strongly accented and/or detached chords, varying tempi and metre, repeating song-like material – went unheard and unresponded to and I often struggled just to be heard. Gradually, there were points where Peter could join and sustain a pulse with me for several beats before returning to the chaotic playing. However, these points often felt like the still eye of a hurricane as the turbulence and sheer volume of Peter's playing made awareness and connection almost impossible. And so, after much deliberation, I first of all removed the cymbal from the room and then, after a six-week summer break, decided to introduce a different way of working where we sat either side of a pair of bongos, using our hands to play. There were several clinical reasons for this. First, it brought the volume level down considerably, which enabled both of us to hear better what was going on in the shared music. Second, I hoped this might enable us to work more easily on essential communication skills such as listening, turn taking, etc. Third, it brought us physically closer, very directly facing each other, which is more relationally demanding for an autistic person but for which I felt Peter was ready.

Here my focus shifted towards a developmental perspective, with particular consideration of autism (see Figure 10.1 point 2, particularly a) and b)). However, this was still being done through the medium and means of the music, as in Figure 10.1, point 1.

Development A

One of the aims I had was to encourage Peter to use his voice interactively in the sessions. Nordoff and Robbins (1977) wrote that 'the more musically communicative an autistic child becomes, the freer he is in response and expression in the therapy situation, and the closer his contact with the therapist(s)' (p.193). The voice is one of our most personal and direct means of spontaneous communication of expression and relationship, and it felt enormously important for Peter to be able to use his voice interactively with me and to be able to develop the possibility of melody and song as a vehicle for creative expression.

Peter had vocalized a little during the goodbye music, but not often, and so, as we sat facing each other across the bongos, I began to use single vocal sounds very directly to him, to try for some vocal response. Peter gradually responded to this, first of all echoing my short 'uh' sounds, which developed into games of exchanging different vowel sounds with me and then 'yes/no' exchanges. During this Peter's monotone inflection became more varied, and there were extended periods of game-playing and shared humour between us – a real development in relation to Peter's autism and general inability to play imaginatively.

Around this time Peter began to pick up on a simple song I'd created around his bongo playing (Figure 10.2) and he used this to create new words within the song structure, first in connection with his playing and then moving on to telling stories about himself, all within the structure of the song.

For the person with autism, very often the only alternatives, both musically and generally, are obsessive rigidity or unstructured chaos. I therefore felt this was an enormous advance for Peter, first in grasping and using a structure, and second, in being able to create words imaginatively which fitted into this – a combination of holding structure flexibly and creatively that people with autism find so hard. He also began through song to express feelings about himself and the things which had happened to him. However, he could only do this indirectly – in the songs and stories he never allowed himself to come to music but took the role of other people, such as the driver of the school bus or other children.

In these roles, he spoke and sang, often in a very punitive way, of what happened to 'Peter' each day, of hating 'Peter', that 'Peter' was waiting in the car park to come to music but that he wouldn't let him, that 'Peter' was crying because he wanted to come, and so on. This was very painful material and it

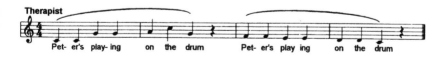

Figure 10.2

was notable that Peter didn't ever allow himself to have the emotion directly but only through the voice of someone else.

After some months of this, at the end of one session, Peter came to the piano and the following musical dialogue ensued, with Peter initially taking the role of 'Sam B', one of the other children in the school (Figure 10.3b). I have transcribed the first few lines of the music to show Peter's ability to relate to structure whilst creating new and relevant words (Figure 10.3a). It is fascinating, in terms of the autistic child's difficulties with understanding self in relation to others, which often results in confusion in grammatical construction, to see how Peter can clearly think of himself in varying ways, both conceptually and semantically – for example, '*Peter* is waiting for *Sam B* to go'; '*Peter* is shouting for *me* to go'; '*Peter's* come to music…did you miss *me?*', where all the highlighted words relate to himself.

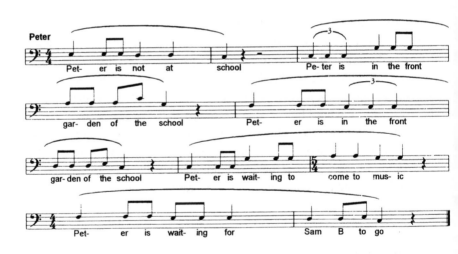

Figure 10.3a

P: Peter is not at home. Peter is in the front garden of the school. Peter is waiting to come to music. Peter is waiting for Sam B to go.

Th: He's waiting outside, waiting to come in; waiting outside, waiting to come in.

P: Peter is shouting at the door for Sam B to go; Peter is shouting for me to go.

Th: Because he wants to come to music himself; because he wants to come to music himself.

(both move to piano)

P: Now Peter's come to music; at *last* Peter's come to music.

Th: At last Peter's come to music.

P: Did you miss me?   – Th: I missed you, Peter.

P: Were you crying for me?   – Th: I was crying for you.

P: And now it's nice to see me.   – Th: It's nice to see you, Peter.

P: Sam B has gone to class 1; Sam B has gone to the classroom.

Th: And Peter came instead, he came to music instead. You're welcome, Peter, at music; you're welcome, Peter, at music. I missed you, I missed you, I missed you at music today.

Figure 10.3b

This was a very poignant moment and I think it shows clearly how vital it is not to define a person in terms of a pathology – for example, autism – but to see everyone we work with as full human beings, with an emotional life and emotional needs. As Jolliffe, herself a young woman with autism, wrote, 'contrary to what people may think, it is possible for an autistic person to feel lonely and to love somebody' (Jolliffe, Lansdown and Robinson 1992, p.14).

Peter continued to work in this way for the rest of the school term. Although noting the advances he had made communicatively in terms of his autism, my focus was now on totally supporting and containing the painful material that he brought, working through song to encourage his fragile emerging sense of self.

On resuming therapy after the six-week summer break, however, Peter did not return to this material and so we again worked purely instrumentally, with bongos, piano and, now, glockenspiel. The glockenspiel had been introduced for a variety of clinical reasons: first, to try to encourage a finer motor control and more awareness in Peter's playing – as any harsh and unfocused playing tended to make the bars bounce off – and, second, to encourage the development of melodic line and phrase. This return to working therapeutically through specific musical aims, as described in Figure 10.1, was to continue for the whole of the next school year.

Development B

Just before the next summer break, one year later, Peter began to make 'Tarzan calls' in the school, and also in many inappropriate places outside as well. As you can imagine, this caused considerable problems and disruption but it was impossible to stop him. After the holidays he began to make these calls throughout the music therapy sessions and I saw no option but to find a way of joining them, in order to try to bring them into some shared musical experience. A challenge indeed!

At first, therefore, I worked to form some kind of pitch relationship with the sounds. After some time, what began to happen was that the last sound of the call began to lengthen and become more pitched, and I worked with this vocally.

After some months of working in this way I became aware, when listening to the tapes of the sessions, that the quality of the end sound of the Tarzan call was changing and I kept finding myself thinking: 'This is sounding more and more like a baby crying.' So, again my focus shifted, and I began to encompass more psychodynamic thoughts, for example concerning regression, containment and countertransference (Figure 10.1, point 3). In the sessions I also began to be more and more aware of my images in relation to this baby and the quality of cries that it made.

Here, as always, the core of the work was in the improvisational musical relationship and I continually worked with the musical qualities I heard, but my understanding of analytic theory was very supportive for me in upholding the very different kinds of music that felt intuitively appropriate at different times, especially when I wasn't sure whether I was hearing anything different from Peter or just imagining qualitative changes in a sound which was really just obsessively and autistically stuck. These apparent changes were very much reflected by the kind of images that came to me during this period. Sometimes, I would feel very affectionate to this crying baby, which, although crying, seemed more 'grizzling' than really upset. I very much had the feeling of being the mother who's moving around, doing other things, while saying 'there there' and feeling very calm and containing and nurturing to this baby, and the music I made reflected this feeling in its consonance, quiet dynamic, often 6/8 metre, clear phrase and structure.

At other times I felt much more distress from Peter – this crying felt much more desolate and might continue for the entire session. When this quality came in the sessions, I often felt I was receiving what it felt like to be the mother who feels desperate, that nothing she can do will soothe this child and stop the crying. Here, in the music, I supported him, still *legato*, with pulse and structure, but often in a more astringent way and in the Phrygian mode. The image in my mind was of saying 'I hear you, I hear how bad it is for you' and being there beside the baby, containing these difficult feelings (cf. Bion 1962).

I felt that my perceptions had been correct concerning the baby quality of Peter's sounds when the first part of the Tarzan call began disappearing and only the last crying sound was left. This wasn't all the time, but quite often we had extended periods of this in the sessions. There was again considerable variety to these sounds, but often a quality of distress and desolation. As time went on, I felt the need to reflect and stay with the painfulness, mirroring this in more detached playing, augmented intervals and dissonance, while, at times, providing a feeling of holding and containment through legato non-verbal vocalizing.

Running in parallel with this 'baby' material, but beginning some time later, Peter introduced strong roaring and vomiting sounds. These were very powerful and intense and I supported them with dissonance and strong non-pulsed music. These sounds had a very powerful effect on me and I felt that Peter was in touch with, and expressing, very strong angry pre-verbal emotions. Again, from a psychotherapeutic understanding, it seemed vital that these were contained and didn't become overwhelming. So, after some time, I deliberately moved from the rather chaotic arhythmic music towards a strong holding pulse, with repeated chords, to ground and hold it all.

These roaring and vomiting sounds became a feature of the work from session to session, alternating with the Tarzan calls and the crying baby sounds. Although I was still working with the musical qualities of Peter's sounds, the thoughts which were very helpful to me here were around issues of the early emotional states of the baby, as discussed by people like Klein, Winnicott and Stern (see Figure 10.1, point 3 and Further Reading).

Holding the tension between thought and creativity is so often the major task of the music therapist. The deliberate introduction of a strong holding pulse and repeated chords to contain Peter's roaring was one of the few times that I consciously *in the moment* used a musical device for a non-musical purpose. My musical style or idiom virtually always occurred as an intuitive and creative response to the musical qualities of Peter at that time, and very rarely as a conscious result of imposing theory from other models.

However, outside of the sessions I found myself constantly monitoring whether this work was meaningful, was communicative. Was Peter just perseverating autistically, absorbed in the sensory aspects of these noises? Was the baby my invention? How could I know what was right? I often felt useless and constantly had to remind myself of the therapeutic necessity and value of not knowing – what Keats (1970) calls 'Negative Capability', the being able to stay in uncertainty 'without any irritable reaching after fact and reason' (p.43).

Here what was crucial was the ability to live in and work with the *musical* relationship, holding the core of the developing work both in creating a musical and emotional environment and in working with particular musical components such as pulse, structure, legato or detached sound, consonance, dissonance, different intervals, as in (Figure 10.1, point 1).

After many weeks of working like this Peter started to make barking noises, and this began to occupy large sections of the sessions. Again, the dilemma continued for me as to whether or not these sounds were perseverative and meaningless or if there was a communicative intent somewhere in it all, and I felt very inadequate as a therapist.

As time went on I began singing about roaring and barking animals, but still with no apparent effect. I tried to think about why dogs barked – is it because they're defensive, angry, frightened? In the session was it to do with a part of Peter that wanted to bite and tear and be angry? I couldn't find a way forward from this and so I continued on, working as before for musical connections and development.

Then, one day, I sang: 'If the dog could speak, what would it say?' And as Peter barked a reply with a clear sense of structure and phrase, it was as if a light had come on for me. I suddenly thought: this dog *is* answering my question but I can't understand it because we speak a different language. *This* is Peter's experience, of constantly trying to communicate with the world around, to understand how other people function and feel, but without success, as if he and they are speaking in foreign languages in which neither understands the other. And so I began to sing 'The dog keeps talking but no one can understand him' and Peter barked and roared with enormous excitement, as if saying: 'She's got there at last!'

This felt so right at the time – that after weeks of struggling with the barking and other vocal sounds, we'd come to some resolution and into some shared communication of how it was for Peter. It was interesting to reflect on the relative effect of words and music in relation to the effectiveness of this intervention – there was a definite response to the words of the first line of Figure 10.4 but an equally significant one to my purely musical change in preparation for my last sung line, with a sense of something very deeply meaningful occurring for Peter both before and after the last sung line.

Recapitulation

Over the following weeks and months we continued to work with this material, and with Peter's instrumental playing, and consolidating and integrating this took us into the final section of our work together. Over the course of the therapy things had changed enormously, and very positively, for Peter in terms of his sense of self, his relationships and how he coped with life in general. So, after consultation with school staff, I decided it was appropriate to move towards ending therapy, which we did in December the following year.

Th: Oh, the dog's talking, but no one can understand him
(P barks loudly)

Oh, the lion's roaring, but no one can understand him
(P roars loudly)

Oh, the angry lion, the angry lion, and the angry dog.
(P continues)

Oh, the angry lion – oh – no one can understand him.

(Therapist changes to piano dynamic/ *legato*; Peter becomes silent)

Th: And no one can understand what it feels like to be Peter.
(suspended moment for both)

Figure 10.4

In our penultimate session together, Peter came in and began to sing 'We wish you a merry Christmas' with much enthusiasm. However, he then began to create his own words within the structure of the song, which, as noted earlier, was quite remarkable in terms of his autism. I was delighted at his pleasure and his evident awareness of the humour of his words and also at a quite extended section where we exchanged animal grunts with each other perfectly in the tempo and flow of the music (Figure 10.5).

It was after this that I had an insight into the Tarzan call: in this seemingly meaningless and perseverative sound was contained, like a dormant seed, all of the issues and difficulties representing the whole of Peter's struggles in the past year. It seemed to me that the choice of the Tarzan call, however unconscious, was amazingly apt – Tarzan calling to his wild animals, which, although still wild, become controllable and his friends, as had Peter's internal 'wild animals'; and the baby, exemplifying the vulnerable, needy aspects of Peter's emotional life, which he was able to acknowledge and accept, and was able to express and share through the baby sounds developed from the call. And in this song the changing focus of my thoughts and clinical aims seemed to come together, in the musical pulse, structure and flexibility found between us (Figure 10.1, point 1), the growth in communicative skills and social interaction (Figure 10.1, point 2), and the acceptance of his 'inner life', in relationship with others, as well as a growing sense of self (Figures 10.1, point 2c and 10.1, point 3).

P: We wish Tarzan a merry Christmas, (repeated several times)
     And a nice hot African summer for Tarzan.
     We wish Tarzan a merry Christmas,
     And a nice hot African summer.
     And we hope Tarzan has a nice summer at Christmas time.
     Good tidings we bring to Tarzan and his wild animals.
     We wish Tarzan a merry Christmas, and a Happy New Year.
     And Tarzan could scream to wish his wild animals at
     Christmas time. (Peter makes Tarzan calls)

Figure 10.5

Th: Peter's wild animals inside.

P: (Animal sounds, continuing)

Th: Here's a wild animal, Peter's wild animal.
      Oh! says Peter's wild animal!
      Oo! says Peter's wild animal!
      Oh! – (we exchange various grunts, vowel sounds and roars,
      all in tempo)
      Oh! says Peter's wild animals inside… (etc.)

Figure 10.5 continued

Coda

So what conclusions does this bring us to in terms of my dilemma? Is the meaning in the music, in the thought, in the symbolism? Does it matter? It seems vital that we, as music therapists, should recognize the power and the experience beyond words that music holds for us all and that, as music therapists, we have something uniquely valuable to offer – rather than just as an adjunct to verbal therapy, music *can* stand on its own, is its own meaning. However, each music therapist also has his or her own unique skills, abilities, experience and understanding to offer to each therapy relationship. Casement (1985) writes: 'When…therapists go rather more "by the patient" and less by the particular theoretical orientation by which they feel supported, it becomes easier to notice when a patient feels out of tune', reminding us that any therapy process will become 'seriously restricted if therapists define themselves out of this possibility in the name of their own chosen orthodoxy' (p.25).

However, perhaps what most enables the therapy process is when we, as therapists, trust and are in tune with ourselves and what we have to offer. Then the dilemma is no longer a dilemma but an embracing of a creative struggle in which we can draw on all of our resources for whatever frees and assists the therapy process at that time, without that process being limited by adherence to a particular model for the model's sake. Only then can client and therapist fully resonate together in creating the music of their own unique relationship.

Glossary

Containment: Bion (1962) introduced the concept of the therapist as 'container'. He parallelled this with early development, when a mother/carer who is emotionally receptive to her baby is able to 'take in', contain and process the raw confused feelings of the baby – particularly those of extreme distress – and then return them to the baby in a modified and manageable form. Through this, the baby has an experience of someone who can make sense of her/his experiences and can then begin to internalize this capacity for her/himself. In therapy the therapist can provide a similar experience of containment and transformation of previously unmanageable and unbearable emotional states for the client.

Countertransference: this refers to the therapist's experience in the session of feelings and images belonging to the client. The therapist 'may be so in tune with his patient's inner world that he finds himself feeling or behaving in a way which he can see, with later understanding, is but an extension of his patient's intrapsychic processes' (Samuels, Shorter and Plaut 1986, p.21). This can give the therapist insight and help to inform the ongoing therapy work.

Exposition/Development/Recapitulation: these are musical terms which describe the sections of classical sonata form.

Frame: the 'therapeutic frame' is built from factors such as regularity in timing, length and frequency of sessions, and clear boundaries in terms of confidentiality and behaviour. This consistency 'provides a safe space with secure foundations' (Gray 1994, p.10) in which the therapy process can take place.

Musical–emotional environment: Nordoff and Robbins (1977) wrote of the need, at particular times, to create for the client 'a musical–emotional environment with which he may feel some affinity...[the therapist's] aim is to communicate with him *as he is*' (p.93). Here the therapist aims to create music that paints a musical portrait of the client, using different idioms and styles to reflect and enhance the emotional qualities perceived in him or her to give the client a new experience of her/himself.

Regression: this involves returning to an earlier stage of development. The theory of regression presupposes that 'infantile stages of development are not entirely outgrown, so that the earlier patterns of behaviour remain available...regression compels the individual to re-experience anxiety appropriate to the stage to which he has regressed' (Rycroft 1968, p.139). Regression can occur in response to life situations – for example, a child returning to bed-wetting or thumb-sucking on the birth of a sibling – and in therapy when early unresolved issues and/or uncontained feelings can be re-experienced and resolved.

References

Ansdell, G. (1995) *Music for Life: Aspects of Creative Music Therapy with Adult Clients.* London: Jessica Kingsley Publishers.

Bion, W. (1962) *Learning from Experience.* London: Heinemann.

Brown, S. (1994) 'Autism and music therapy – is change possible, and why music?' *Journal of British Music Therapy 8,*1, 15–25.

Casement, P. (1985) *On Learning from the Patient.* London and New York: Tavistock Publications.

Gray, A. (1994) *An Introduction to the Therapeutic Frame.* London and New York: Routledge.

John, D. (1992) 'Towards music psychotherapy.' *Journal of British Music Therapy 6,* 1, 10–12.

Jollife, T., Lansdown, R. and Robinson, C. (1992) 'Autism: A personal account' *Communication 26,* 3, 12–19.

Keats, J. (1970) 'To George and Tom Keats, 21, 27(?) December 1817.' In R.Gittings (ed) *Letters of John Keats – A New Selection.* London, Oxford and New York: Oxford University Press.

Nordoff, P. and Robbins, C. (1971) *Therapy in Music for Handicapped Children.* London and New York: Gollancz.

Nordoff, P. and Robbins, C. (1977) *Creative Music Therapy.* New York: The John Day Company.

Rycroft, C. (1968) *A Critical Dictionary of Psychoanalysis.* London: Penguin Books

Samuels, A., Shorter, B. and Plaut, F. (1986) *A Critical Dictionary of Jungian Analysis.* London and New York: Routledge.

Trevarthen, C., Aitken, K., Papoudi, D. and Robarts J. (1996) *Children with Autism (2nd Edition).* London: Jessica Kingsley Publishers.

Wing, L. (1993) *Autistic Continuum Disorders: An Aid to Diagnosis.* London: National Autistic Society.

Further Reading

Hinshelwood, R.D. (1991) *A Dictionary of Kleinian Thought (2nd Edn).* London: Free Association Books.

Stern, D.N. (1990) *The Interpersonal World of the Infant.* London: Basic Books.

Winnicott, D.W. (1990) *The Maturational Processes and the Facilitating Environment.* London: Karnac Books.

PART THREE

Neurology

CHAPTER 11

'Singing My Life, Playing My Self'
Music Therapy in the Treatment
of Chronic Neurological Illness

Wendy Magee

Music therapy orientation

This chapter presents the results of a research study which examined the experience of music therapy for individuals living with chronic neurological illness. Particular focus was given to comparing the use of unfamiliar improvised music in clinical improvisations with the use of pre-composed familiar songs. The aim was to determine the differences in each of these in music therapy. From the research findings, recommendations for clinical applications will be drawn which encompass different aspects of the human condition and the experience of living with neurological illness.

My clinical music therapy orientation reflects my own cultural experience of having trained in Australia and then moving to work in Britain, in that I combine the use of songs and clinical improvisation as appropriate to an individual's needs. My theoretical orientation draws from neuro-behavioural frameworks of practice – that is, I consider not only an individual's psychosocial needs but give equal consideration to their neuro-cognitive functioning. For example, when working with individuals with cognitive impairments, I interpret musical events considering aspects of functioning such as memory, initiation, conceptual and reasoning skills, perception, and the ability to plan, sequence and carry out an intended action. In doing so I gain an understanding of the meaning musical events hold for an individual who is cognitively impaired and how his or her responses may best be interpreted. However, in addition to neuro-cognitive functioning, an individual's emotional needs are also given weight. In this study clinical supervision from a psychodynamic perspective gave alternative interpretations of the musical events. These interpretations aided in facilitating a fuller understanding of the individuals' complex emotional needs.

The participants[1] in this study were hospitalized with Multiple Sclerosis. Multiple Sclerosis is a chronic progressive neurological disease caused by the widespread breakdown of the covering of the nerve fibres throughout the brain and spinal cord, resulting in motor disturbances, sensory disturbances and changes in cognition (Walton 1977). It is characterized by periods of relapse and remission. Multiple Sclerosis is the most common non-traumatic neurological illness affecting young and middle-aged adults (Rao 1986). At present, the cause of the disease remains undetermined and its course is variable between minimal effects to severe and chronic disability. The available treatment tends to be symptomatic or preventative in nature and individuals cannot be given accurate prognoses. Many people with Multiple Sclerosis experience cognitive dysfunction and research indicates that large numbers experience subcortical dementia (Mahler and Benson 1990). The severest possible physical symptoms experienced may include ataxia or paralysis impairing nearly all voluntary and functional movement, loss of speech, the inability to swallow and extreme fatigue. Emotional responses and reactions are as individual and dynamic as the disease course itself but dramatic changes in physical abilities and levels of independence affect self-concept and identity. The participants who took part in this study were either living in hospital or living at home and attending a day centre. All had moderate to severe physical disabilities as a consequence of Multiple Sclerosis. Results of neuropsychological tests were also drawn upon to reveal each individual's level of cognitive involvement. This varied across individuals from mild cognitive impairment to a moderate level of subcortical dementia. All the participants were physically able to use musical instruments, using one hand or arm, and all were able to communicate verbally. All were wheelchair dependent. The age range was 29 to 52 years of age.

1   The term 'participants' is used rather than 'research subjects' as fitting to the qualitative methodology employed in this enquiry.

Clinical material

Methods of application and descriptions of music material

Within this study the clinical application of two different types of music were compared. These were pre-composed familiar songs of the participant's choice or unfamiliar improvised music within turn taking or clinical improvisations. The music differed in essential aspects: the songs possessed familiar musical structures and drew on long-term memory, whereas the improvised material was unfamiliar, involved shorter-term memory skills and could vary in structure, such as the familiarity of harmonic progressions or tonality used. In the early part of the data collection period sessions used exclusively improvisation or songs within any one session, alternated on a weekly basis.[2] As the therapy process developed and familiarity with both activities increased, participants were encouraged to choose which type of music or activity they wished to use at the start of their session. In this way, participants were encouraged to control the process through choice, making as much as possible, and clinical application remained patient focused. All music used in the sessions was live.

Song-based techniques have been described elsewhere in the music therapy literature with a variety of clinical populations for different therapeutic purposes (Bailey 1984; Martin 1991; O'Callaghan 1995, 1996; Whittal 1991). The song-based sessions involved singing and playing songs or pre-composed pieces of the participant's choice. It was essential that the songs held personal meaning to the individuals and that they had chosen the songs themselves. In the song sessions the focus was on singing and playing the songs chosen, although discussion of themes, personal associations and reminiscences about the songs may have also been stimulated and included as part of the therapy process. Early in the therapy process in song-based sessions styles of music or songs of personal relevance to the individual were determined. In conjunction with the participant, the therapist located songs of the participant's choice or songs which held particular meaning for the participant. Hence verbal material was central to this part of the process. Over the sessions the therapist built up a full repertoire of an individual's preferred songs.

---

2   This design was adopted for research purposes and does not reflect the author's typical application of clinical methods.

Once this personal repertoire was established, the therapist drew on the individual's personal repertoire to offer song choices, ensuring that a range of moods and themes were always provided in the song choices offered. This allowed the participant the opportunity to set the mood or theme through the music. The songs chosen by participants in this way were played by the therapist on piano or guitar, or by the participant on the autoharp with some assistance. The participant was offered pitched and unpitched percussion and strumming instruments to play to accompany the songs. The participant chose whether or not the words were sung by either her or himself and/or by the therapist. After each song there was time for any verbal or non-verbal reflection, depending on behavioural and emotional responses to the music. If there was a particularly emotional response to the song, this was acknowledged by the therapist with opportunity for discussion if the participant wished. As the therapist developed an understanding of how an individual interacted with their songs, that is, what emotions were elicited, and what meaning and associations were held with a particular song, the songs could be drawn on more intuitively by the therapist. This reflected the development of the therapeutic relationship.

Improvisation sessions involved presenting to the participant a range of tuned and untuned percussion instruments, small strumming instruments and electric piano.[3] Exploration was encouraged either independently, or in turn-taking activities with the therapist. A great deal of time needed to be spent ensuring that instruments met the physical limitations of the participants, who had varying degrees of physical problems. Instruments sometimes needed to be adapted or physical aids brought to the session to aid in playing. Exploration in this way enabled discovery of the musical qualities and ranges of the chosen instruments. Turn-taking activities also served the purpose of extending and developing individuals' use of musical components through imitation. Active participation in spontaneous improvisations was also facilitated in exploration. If the individual did not engage spontaneously in this way, the improvisations may have been more structured – for example, on a theme suggested by the participant or therapist. If thematically based, concrete subjects such as a style of music may have been drawn upon, or more abstract themes drawn from the participant's

3   The upright piano available in the treatment room was inaccessible for participants due to the size of wheelchairs and the nature of the physical disabilities. For this reason, electric piano was used.

verbal material, such as relationships. Mostly, improvisations were purely instrumental. However, occasionally, they involved both instruments and the participant's vocalizations. One participant who considered music therapy a place to sing his songs was encouraged to improvise vocally over a simple and familiar tonic/subdominant/dominant harmony. Due to the anxiety he felt about singing without the structure of words and a familiar melody, time was spent preparing him for this vocal improvisation through breathing and vocal warm-up exercises.

Mostly after improvisation activity, time was provided for non-verbal reflection or spontaneous discussion on associations, feelings or thoughts aroused by the sounds and music being made. Once again, this depended on emotional, behavioural and musical responses within the improvisation. Verbal reflection was not considered essential within the process, however, participants often spontaneously started to discuss their music making. It was acknowledged that responses had taken place implicitly within the musical structures and the interactive musical relationship. The purpose or role of improvisation was not explained or described to the individual prior to music therapy as the aim of this research was to allow the participants' own experiences to emerge within the data collection.

Relevance of therapist's musical role

The therapist's musical role depended on the type of activity used in the session. Even when the therapist's musical role was central to the music making, participants were encouraged to remain actively involved in all aspects of the music within the session.

For example, the participants' choice was central to their own instrumental sounds, the therapist's instrument and whether or not lyrics should be sung. Within song sessions, although it was the therapist who played the melody and harmony, individuals were invited to sing. It was noted that most often this happened spontaneously. Additionally, each participant was offered a non-pitched percussion instrument to play during songs. Non-pitched instruments were offered so that individuals did not feel pressured to play a melody but, instead, could tap a rhythm or pulse. The types of instruments offered included drums with beaters, bongos and a range of African shakers, rattles and drums. Even when a participant chose 'just to listen', it was observed that he or she was motivated to respond in some small way, such as tapping his or her fingers on the wheelchair tray. Within the song sessions the musical material relied heavily on the therapist.

To enhance the interactive aspect of the songs' activities, it was important that the therapist took some aspect of the music from the individual. This may have been rhythm from the individual's playing, tempo from the individual's breathing rate or pitch from the individual's vocalizations. The aim of using songs was to draw on familiar musical structures to facilitate emotional expression and facilitate reflection on the past, the changes that had occurred for the individual and the impact of these changes on the present.

Within the clinical improvisations the therapist drew from the individual's musical sounds and structures, reflecting, developing and extending these. The focus was on non-verbal interaction within musical components. The therapist usually worked from the piano in improvisation sessions but may have used flute, autoharp or pitched percussion instruments such as the bass xylophone or alto metallophone. Frequently, the therapist used her voice at some stage during most improvisations to sing a melody line. The therapist's musical role was predominantly to give a musical framework or structure to the participant's musical sounds. For example, one participant's music usually consisted of variations of a syncopated rhythm of:

Her variations on this rhythm were, at times, complex, such as:

and:

The therapist's music most often gave chordal harmonic support in longer time values to these rhythms, occasionally reflecting part of the quaver and crochet syncopation. It was important to reflect the participant's rhythms in some way in order for her to have felt 'met' in the music. This participant responded to these rhythmic interchanges and, if she did not hear them, would stop playing suddenly and ask: 'Have we stopped?'[4] It was, therefore, important to give her some reflection of her rhythms without merely imitating the intensity of her driving rhythms. The aim of using clinical

---

4   As this participant was blind, she was unable to use any visual cues to orientate her to events. She therefore relied heavily on aural cues.

improvisation was to encourage exploration through sound and non-verbal interaction within a supportive and boundaried environment.

In the data collected individuals reported that within the improvisations they experienced the music to be more interactive. For example, participants reported feeling a more dynamic relationship with the therapist through such terms as 'following', 'leading' and 'mirroring'. One participant reflected after an improvisation in which she played the metallophone and the windchimes with the therapist at the piano:

> Well I think we're sort of mirroring the other one. When you were playing sort of softer I was playing more down here (indicates section of metallophone). And I was sort of playing up here (taps bass notes of metallophone). And the windchimes as well (plays some sounds on the windchimes) ... I was playing and we were sort of mirroring each other, so when you were playing softer, I was trying to play softer, and that when I get loud you got louder on the piano. Yeah ...'interaction'.

Role of the music in the therapeutic process

Using techniques drawn from grounded theory methodology and triangulation with multiple-data sources, it emerged that songs and improvisation held very different roles in the music therapy process. Unfamiliar improvised music within clinical improvisations provided a more dynamic sense of interaction than the techniques involving familiar songs. As improvisation was unique for each of the participants to the relationship with the therapist, as opposed to other relationships in their lives, it possessed a potential which, for some of the participants, was intense and ultimately threatening. Although familiar music also had some interactive qualities, these were not as subtle or varied as those for improvisation.

In addition to the interactive potential with improvised music, the physical involvement in playing instruments was significant in participants' experiences. For example, individuals frequently commented on how well or poorly they had handled an instrument and how their physical manner of playing an instrument differed from previous sessions. Also, extreme fatigue inhibited the ability to sustain playing for some individuals or individuals may have had difficulty controlling their movements due to ataxia. These problems meant that playing instruments involved physical negotiation between the body and the environment. This connected the experience of improvisation to larger issues relating to the illness process. However, individuals had difficulty finding meaning in improvising, sensing it as something at which they were not skilled. This raised feelings about independence and dependence which also related to feelings of identity concerning the changes experienced as a result of illness. For example, one man who had played guitar prior to his illness reflected on the change in his skills after an improvisation in which he had strummed a guitar tuned to an open chord of D major: 'It's a bit annoying when you can't play guitar ... like I used to.'

As clinical improvisation involved physically manipulating instruments, early on in therapy it was experienced as a more physical achievement rather than a musical act or interpersonal activity, particularly for individuals who had difficulty grasping or maintaining a grasp on an instrument or beater, difficulty reaching out to play an instrument, or could not gain any sense of controlled movement. All these aspects affected what sounds an individual gained from the instruments and what control he or she achieved over components such as dynamics, intensity, rhythm, pitch and duration.

However, other themes were also prominent in the experience of improvisation, particularly that of 'interaction/relationship'. It was through the interactive phenomenon, heightened within clinical improvisation, that individuals had their attempts to physically interact with the environment supported and reflected by the therapist. Through the process of mutual music making within clinical improvisation, individuals were able to achieve altered sensations of ability, independence, skill, achievement and success. Dramatic shifts occurred resulting in altered self-concepts. Hence individuals attained more 'able' identities through the act of music making.

For example, one woman frequently presented at the start of sessions in a withdrawn manner, verbally giving negative views of herself in a quiet and monotonous voice. Her responses within verbal interactions were delayed or absent. She found it difficult to make choices and her movements were small, clumsy, unconfident and limited to a small area within the range of her wheelchair tray. In improvisations she played a range of instruments which necessitated her to reach outside of the usual range around her with great precision. She played energetically for prolonged periods of time, alternating between instruments rapidly and with accuracy. Changes in her levels of arousal were visible in her facial gestures, range of physical movements and spontaneity of her musical interactions. After improvisations she reported feeling more aroused. This was supported by the spontaneity of her verbal interactions and her tone of voice, which showed greater variety in pitch and volume than prior to improvisation. She reported the following with regard to how she felt about her improvising. 'I think it was good ... sounded alright ... as if we knew what we both were playing ... it was very corresponding. It sort of roused me. Yes. It sounded like a *professional* musician playing ... Maybe I was thinking I *knew* how to play these instruments.'

In this example the concept of 'interaction' emerges in the word 'corresponding', which she used to describe her feeling of being met in the music. This led on to her sense of 'skill', which is indicated through her feelings of being 'professional' and expressions of confidence in her playing. These expressions of skill differed dramatically from the regular negative statements she made about herself in her verbal material at the start of sessions. This indicated that through the experience of improvisation her feelings of skill increased, in turn affecting her feelings about herself.

It was found that pre-composed music held a very different role in the therapy process. Because of the associations held with songs to events, people and places throughout an individual's life, songs represented old friends who had seen through good and bad times alike. Individuals had not been deserted by 'their' songs as they had been deserted by friends and family. Songs held a particular meaning which was highly individual. In this way they could be used to communicate something personal about the individual in an explicit or implicit way. The words and messages embodied within songs and the emotional qualities within the musical structures of the songs also served to communicate something for or about the individual. This may have been either to the therapist or to a significant other from the past, present or future. This aspect of familiar music also enabled it to express a deeper 'real' self or, alternatively, be used to mask feelings which were too difficult for the individual to have openly acknowledged in words or music.

Songs also supported individuals in their coping strategies. In dealing with their long-term, ongoing, progressive illness, a range of coping styles and mechanisms were revealed in individuals' behaviours and use of music. A process emerged from the data indicating that individuals initially identified a feeling or emotional state during the musical experience and then, according to whether they felt this was an acceptable way of being or not, either adopted a 'Coping Front' or moved to a state of 'Barriers Down' (Magee 1998). Many condition variables affected this process, such as feelings of threat, control, trying to make sense of their illness, insight, feelings of hope and the degree of change experienced as a consequence of illness.

Familiar songs allowed individuals to feel the more difficult feelings which they otherwise may have been denying. In requesting a specific song of personal meaning, individuals brought certain emotional states to the fore within the sessions in their music. For example, a song may have been known to stimulate for a participant more vulnerable feelings and issues such as loss, love or yearning for the past. The feelings stimulated by a song would have been established by the therapist early in the therapy process. In requesting this song an individual was not just requesting the musical structures, such as the melody and harmony, but the implicit personal meanings and emotions of that song. For example, one young man who frequently presented with a brash front often requested a favourite rock ballad when he felt safe enough to explore a more vulnerable side to himself. It was established in an early session that, for him, the song had the power to 'bring a tear to my eye'. Later, he reflected on the loss of independence and everything that was important to him, expressions which were stimulated by this song and what it represented to him. Individuals each had their personal repertoire of songs, hence the familiar songs used differed for each individual. The use of familiar songs allowed individuals to move in and out of their coping strategies at a pace which they controlled. For example, one participant alternated the pop songs 'All Cried Out' and 'The Only Way Is Up'. The first of these she identified on occasions as representing how she felt, trying to cope with her illness. At other times she emphatically insisted that the latter represented her personal goal – up and out of her wheelchair and the hospital. In the therapist gaining an understanding of what particular songs represented to individuals it was possible to support them within the music – that is, implicitly – or, if appropriate, to extend this into words – that is, explicitly. However, it was within the music that the process took place.

Evaluation and interpretation of clinical material

Within this study, data was collected from multiple sources. The main data was collected in the form of focused interviews with the research participants during and after individual music therapy sessions. These interviews were recorded and transcribed by the therapist. Additional data was drawn from participants' musical, behavioural and verbal material documented in session evaluation notes by the therapist immediately after sessions by transcribing audio recordings of the sessions. Data was collected in this way over a six-month period for each participant.

The data was analysed using a modified form of grounded theory. Grounded theory is defined as:

...one that is inductively derived from the study of the phenomenon it represents. That is, it is discovered, developed, and provisionally verified through systematic data collection and analysis of data pertaining to that phenomenon. Therefore, data collection, analysis, and theory stand in reciprocal relationship with each other. (Strauss and Corbin 1990, p.23)

Using this method, themes emerged from the verbal material which were central to the participants' experience of music therapy as it related to their lives.

Clinical material was evaluated immediately after each session by transcribing audio recordings of the session. Musical material from the clinical improvisations was either roughly transcribed using musical notation or described in words. Particular focus was given to changes in individuals' stereotypical musical material and also to key moments of musical interaction. These two particular aspects were focused upon as individuals presented with 'typical' musical material, which may have been due to any combination of cognitive, physical or psychosocial factors. Furthermore, moments of key musical interactions were important to note to determine whether these differed from verbal interactions, particularly in terms of defence mechanisms. Individuals often were well defended with coping strategies in their verbal material, therefore it was essential to examine whether interactions in their musical material were less defended.

For example, one individual each week chose to play the same drum, on which he knew he could elicit the sound he wanted. His musical material was stereotypically an unfaltering, non-interactive pulse at a fairly steady dynamic. A combination of cognitive, emotional and physical factors appeared to contribute to this. Certainly, his physical abilities caused him great difficulty in achieving intentional and controlled movements, his cognitive problems caused difficulty with unfamiliar or abstract tasks and psychodynamic supervision suggested that he was hesitant to allow himself to build a relationship with another. It was important, therefore, to note any changes in his musical sounds and interactions which may have indicated change, development or evidence of musical behaviour transcending the physical and the conscious realms.

All behavioural responses to both the songs and improvisations were also documented accurately. Behavioural responses prior to or at the start of the session were compared with those during or at the end of the session.

Additionally, relevant verbal material from the session was transcribed. Themes within the verbal material were noted in order to make between-session comparisons and examine any emerging patterns. The therapist also noted any reactions of her own within sessions or in response to transcribing the notes, which she took to clinical supervision to examine issues of transference.

To ensure trustworthiness of the analyses, triangulation was achieved on several levels. Validation of the clinical process and, particularly, the improvisational material was gained through clinical supervision. The clinical supervisor was a music therapist whose theoretical stance was based in psychotherapeutic theory and, therefore, differed from the therapist/ researcher's. This served to offer alternative interpretations of the clinical material from the therapist's neuro-behavioural interpretations. An independent auditor familiar with both behavioural and psychodynamic practices triangulated the analyses made of the verbal transcripts. Analyses and interpretations of clinical material were also triangulated with other members of the multidisciplinary team at the hospital – that is, physio- therapists, occupational therapists and nursing staff. In this way a complex picture was built of the individual and verified from different angles.

Although these methods reflect a research methodology and approach, there are many relevant aspects for the clinician in the practical setting. Individuals with neurological illness present with complex needs. These include any combination of emotional, social, neuropsychological, physical, biographical and spiritual factors. For example, when working with an individual's moderate subcortical dementia, the clinician may be faced with a person who is extremely verbal due to both emotional coping mechanisms and cognitive problems. An individual with frontal lobe lesions may present as verbally disinhibited, firing many verbal questions and statements in a non-interactive way. Attention deficits may mean that engagement in musical activity lasts for a very short duration only, with sudden verbal interruptions. The intensity and intimacy of music making may also be perceived as a threatening activity to someone who is trying to cope emotionally with progressive chronic illness. For such individuals, coping mechanisms are often firmly in place for reasons of emotional survival. Hence the triangulation ensured for research purposes in this study reflect the processes which the clinician may follow to meet such complexities in the real world for validation of clinical interpretations.

Returning to actual clinical examples, the following extracts from sessional and interview data revealed emerging themes of the music therapy experience.

The physical impact of playing and singing was prominent in the music therapy experience. For example, one man who had previously played music found that he knew what he wanted to do musically but was not physically able to enact this, which affected his feelings of skill: 'Well because I can play … play … bash the drum or something, but I can't really control my hands enough to get a proper rhythm.'

In a later session the same participant became really frustrated by his physical problems in playing. In the following extract he was commentating on how his playing of a light-weight maraca did not depict the pulse he was trying to control in his music. The sound he achieved with this instrument through his physical interaction with it put into sound his gross uncontrolled movements. He stated: 'I can't play … I shake like that (picks up maraca and shakes with ataxic arm movements). It's not exactly music is it? To do that?'

From these examples, concepts such as 'control', 'failure' and 'skill' started to emerge as relating to the physical experience of music therapy. It was found that individuals monitored their physical abilities through playing instruments, and this phenomenon was entitled 'Physical monitoring' as part of a larger process entitled 'Illness monitoring' (Magee 1998). Through this process, individuals were able to monitor even small changes in their physical functioning. For some participants, the continual search for physical improvements appeared to dominate their experience of the improvising, acting as a barrier to reaching any deeper levels of meaning. This was particularly the case early on in therapy. For example, one woman chose the theme of 'going home' on which to improvise. This was a particularly emotive issue for her as it was her central goal which drove her day-to-day existence. The improvisation was especially expressive, in which the participant chose the windchimes and a hand drum. The therapist used the piano in order to give harmonic and melodic structure to the pulse which the participant tapped out, playing a melody in octaves which gradually expanded out in a broad, rising melody. In the latter part of the improvisation the therapist improvised vocally, singing 'Going home'. There was little eye contact as the participant tapped the pulse and used the windchimes for colour at poignant moments, particularly at the very end. Despite the expressiveness of the music within this improvisation, however, she reported:

... the improvising gives me a good chance to use my right hand, which for so long was just there. You know, I couldn't use it (plays drum) ... I mean I love the windchimes (plays windchimes) ... and using my right arm on the drum's great as well, because (hits drum) you know I could never have done anything like that even when I first came to your music sessions. My arm's ... you know it was a case of get it down and keeping it...

From this example a sense is gained of how individuals made comparisons over time with regard to their physical abilities. If there was positive change experienced, the experience of playing resulted in heightened feelings of achievement and success. However, individuals often did not experience 'positive' change and, instead 'played how they were'. This resulted, at times, in a reinforcement of a 'disabled' identity. Illness monitoring was also noted to occur within song-based activities by individuals monitoring any changes in the quality, volume or breath control in their singing, and also in the ability to recall the words to songs. These phenomena were entitled 'Vocal monitoring' and 'Cognitive monitoring' respectively as part of the subcategory 'Illness monitoring' (Magee 1998).

The physical involvement of music therapy therefore linked in to concepts of 'Identity'. The following example comes much later within the therapy process for the male participant already cited. This man found his physical disabilities immensely frustrating in every situation throughout his day and, also, in how his disabilities restricted his whole lifestyle. In this example he is reflecting immediately after an improvisation which he felt expressed the power and control he was no longer able to enact physically on his environment in any way. Within this improvisation he played an unfaltering pulse with his one functional hand on a large hand drum at a fairly constant dynamic. This was typical of his playing. Around this pulse the therapist played a modal melody in octaves. Initially, the music was sparse but moved constantly to his pulse. As he suddenly quickened his pulse, the music became faster. However, he was unable to physically sustain this tempo and fell back to playing in half-time, skipping every second beat. The therapist's music continued with his intended tempo and the intensity of the dynamics he reached. Immediately afterwards he stated:

It sounded good! ... I liked it – it was very good music ... my beating the tambourine, and your counterpoint music, was very good. Well you were playing the bass bits on there – a very very aggressive bass. And me bashing the tambourine as well. That was aggressive ... Aggressive music was coming out between the two of us ... That was a very good Beethoven improvisation we were doing together. The '1812' bang bang on the tambourine etcetera. Excellent with the piano doing some Holst 'Planets' and that sort of thing.

MT: So what purpose did that serve for you today?

I don't know – after talking about me not being cared for ... and that sort of thing ... it just proved that I can *do* it, you know, and we *did* it – it was pretty good music we did today. Proving I can play pretty good music as well. I wish we could write it up because it was just brilliant music!

His description highlights key concepts relating to 'Identity': ability, independence, achievement, ownership and success. Concepts relating to the interactive nature of improvisation were also central to his experience however. Furthermore, he reflected how the perceived meaning within the improvisation was enhanced through association on an emotional level with pre-composed music.

However, improvisation did not stimulate such processes for all the participants. One of the participants never really engaged in the improvisational activities. He explained why his particular songs were so important for him, alluding to the relationship they held over time. The songs which held special meaning for him were romantic ballads of the 1940s to 1960s, such as 'Ol' Man River' and 'What a Wonderful World':

I'm sure that human beings ... when he sings, he must identify himself with some spot in his life. It must do, well it does do for me. It's all interwoven into your life. These songs are interwoven into my life. Into my experiences ... as a matter of fact, life is a programme ... a programme of what songs go along with you at that particular time. At every stage of your life, there will be some songs that will accompany you. They will be with you. Forever. Forever.

For another participant, particular songs spanned the past, the present and into the future as well. He had one particular song, 'Drive' (written by Ric Ocasek and performed by 'The Cars'), which held great personal meaning and to which he alluded in the following extract. However, he also reflected on what role songs in general played within his life and therapy:

All of my life bends around music. One piece in my head can symbolize somewhere I've been to. With the songs I'm singing parts of my life ...

reliving a part of my life ... I like to see what comes in the future with it as well. That music will never die for me.

Songs also served to aid individuals in their coping strategies. Coping strategies helped individuals manage the emotional effects of living with chronic incurable illness and increased the sense of control. Individuals often revealed a range of strategies which were grouped together under the subcategory 'Coping front'. For example, one of the participants presented in and outside of sessions with an incessant coping front. This participant revealed one such coping strategy verbally in the following extract. He was referring here to the act of singing songs in general, rather than in reference to any one particular song:

Because I don't want down. I (pause) don't come off the same level in my experiences of happiness. I'm happy when I'm singing ... It's unnatural to be unhappy. And that's quite true. (Emphatically) *It is unnatural to be unhappy* ... I don't get sad about it, because you mustn't let the negative ... depression is a very negative thing, and it will break your heart, and the opposite is joy, and that will lift you up ... you've got to be on that side of life all the time...

Within sessions this participant had a small repertoire of favourite songs, such as 'Ol' Man River', 'Some Enchanted Evening' and 'Autumn Leaves'. These were typically emotive within their musical components – that is, slower tempi, rich harmonies, expressive melodies, sustained time values – but lyrically covered a variety of themes – that is, love, hardship, reflection. His verbal descriptions of 'happiness' did not match the music he longed for and loved to sing in every session. It was difficult to ascertain the particular meaning the songs held for him as any exploration seemed to threaten him and resulted in him maintaining a 'coping front'. Within one of the later sessions, however, he revealed that the associations held over his lifespan with the songs matched the deeper emotional experience of his life, which he fought so hard to keep hidden. For the first time, he identified that the songs were not 'happy' and he related the songs to his own feelings. It appeared that although he could not allow himself to feel these more difficult feelings, through singing his 'sad' songs he was able to sing how he felt. In this way the songs helped him to drop his coping front and move to a state of 'Barriers Down', albeit through song. In the following example he reflected on his particular songs, named already, which he frequently requested to sing in sessions:

...they are all sad songs ... they're all about sadness. And sadness in love. And you've got to feel a bit like that to sing them. You've got to feel like that. You've got to ... *be* that way to sing it. Every song that I sing, is sad, I can't help it. I guess there isn't any song I don't find sad. Like, I s'pose, my life makes it sad. (Long pause) Yes, I guess all songs get to the bottom of me ... the reason they all feel sad, is my life I s'pose (laughs with awkwardness). Yeah, it's a *lack of love* (emphatically). I couldn't sing a song that wasn't sad. Maybe it's me protesting the lack of love. Well, I know it is. Yeah, that's how when I look back on my life, it is all these songs.

Relation of practice to theory

Although music therapy has a great deal to offer in the emotional and psychosocial issues identified for this population, to date there exists very little literature suggesting music therapy is widely used with people with Multiple Sclerosis. Lengdobler and Kiessling (1989) described work with Multiple Sclerosis patients, exploring themes around disability, uncertainty, anxiety, depression and loss of self-esteem, using minimally structured improvisations in group therapy. Very different recommendations for the clinical application of music therapy are made elsewhere however. Work with individuals with advanced Multiple Sclerosis showing considerable subcortical dementia and no functional movement strongly recommended the use of familiar music. These recommendations were grounded in an understanding of individuals' cognitive abilities, drawing on neuro-behavioural models (O'Callaghan and Brown 1989; O'Callaghan and Turnbull 1987, 1988). The techniques show how to actively engage individuals who would otherwise be prevented from doing so due to the severity of physical and cognitive disabilities.

The group of participants in this study had varying degrees of physical and cognitive disabilities. The findings presented here reflect that the clinical application in music therapy of both familiar pre-composed music and improvisation has a role to play in meeting individuals' physical and psychosocial needs. It was not enough to consider only cognitive or emotional aspects as the individuals' physical needs were central to their experience.

In examining the literature pertaining to chronic illness, it is revealed that music therapy can indeed offer important clinical intervention. Concepts emerged in the data which were directly affected by the specific application of music therapy techniques. The physical impact of chronic neurological illness has been noted to be central to the individual's experience, as 'when illness brings about a failed body ... the foundations of existence are shaken' (Corbin and Strauss 1987, p.252). When an individual is unable to carry out even the smallest task associated with some aspect of the self, there is a loss of wholeness and of self-identity. These concepts of 'self' and 'identity' occur repeatedly in the literature pertaining to how chronically ill individuals cope with the enormous change and progressive loss experienced through illness (Brooks and Matson 1987; Charmaz 1987; Conrad 1987; Corbin and Strauss 1987; Robinson 1988). When identity is threatened, the individual needs to be able to transcend the body, to come to terms with their losses and build a new conception of 'self' around their limitations. Charmaz (1987), however, identifies that individuals living with chronic illness gradually scale down their self-expectations and that this results in the identity of a 'salvaged self'. The struggle for those profoundly disabled through chronic illness in realizing a preferred identity can never be underestimated. This is particularly so for the individual who has become so immersed and isolated as a consequence of illness that they cannot readily claim other identities in the external world.

Life review is also a significant feature for the individual living with a life-threatening condition (Butler and Lewis 1982). More recently, this has been termed within chronic illness research as 'biographical work'. This can be defined as servicing one's own life through review, maintenance, repair and alteration, aiding an individual's adaptation to the changes which have taken place for them (Corbin and Strauss 1987). Such reviews include various types of imagery examining the past, present and future. This includes what is described as 'identity reconstitution' or reintegrating one's identity into a new concept of wholeness, discovering new and unused aspects of the self. Others play a crucial role in this process through validating the individual's performance and thus reinforcing the individual's reconstructed identity.

Within this study participants revealed that music therapy provided opportunities to challenge the 'disabled' identity which had developed as a consequence of chronic illness. Furthermore, through the interactive nature of improvisation, the therapist provided the 'performance validation' which has been described as necessary for reintegrating one's identity into a 'new concept of wholeness' (Corbin and Strauss 1987).

Concepts such as 'identity' and 'self' have been identified as central to the individual's music therapy process in palliative care also, as 'we sing and play what we are' (Aldridge 1995). However, the individual living with chronic neurological illness often is not dealing with the 'acute crisis' of dying but of living and managing the progressive and long-term nature of their disabilities. For this reason, there are additional psychosocial factors to consider in the treatment of chronic illness. Songs helped to meet such additional needs through supporting individuals in the coping strategies adopted to deal with the emotional impact of their illness. This has been noted already in the use of song-based techniques with hospitalized cancer patients (Bailey 1984). Within the study reported here, although individuals could not verbally explore or acknowledge their more difficult feelings, they could indeed 'sing how they were'. In this way pre-composed music facilitated important emotional work.

The properties of association and relationship over time held by songs give them enormous potential for facilitating the biographical work which has been described as being so important for individuals with chronic illness. Previously, this technique has been described as 'musical life review' (Bright 1986).

However, it is disputed here that using songs for this purpose is an end in itself. Within this research it was often the first step of a deeper process, or a way of building the therapeutic relationship. In this way the use of songs is not merely remedial but may indeed be used more psychodynamically to address deeper and more difficult emotional issues. Participants did not only relay previous experiences to songs. They also related issues which were central to their current existence to the themes, feelings and memories which gave songs their meaning. Participants spoke of the future in connection to their songs. This is highly significant for the individual living with degenerative illness, for whom the future is unknown in every aspect of their existence.

General benefits

The findings of this study suggest that when geared to the individual's needs, there is a role for the combined use of clinical improvisation and pre-composed songs in the clinical application of music therapy for people living with chronic degenerative neurological illness.

A critical issue for the music therapist with this population is the way in which music may be used in maintaining impenetrable coping defences and how to work with them. The therapist must question the purpose of such coping strategies, considering that these are in place for emotional survival. Furthermore, by developing an understanding, the therapist may not be so dismissive of an individual's wish to stay with the use of pre-composed material and, instead, adapt the use of music accordingly.

The concept of control emerged as a fundamental property of the strategies individuals used to cope with the emotional responses to their illness. 'Control' has been identified previously as a mechanism for maintaining self-esteem. Charmaz (1987) reflects that in chronic illness 'coping' is achieved through controlling one's identity and, in doing so, one feels successful due to the 'front' maintained to the outside world. Health psychology research indicates that social interactions are influential in reinforcing the individual's perception of 'coping' or 'managing' (Brooks and Matson 1987). It was evident that, for the individuals in this study, there were few mechanisms available for coping due to the extent to which chronic illness had resulted in isolation and disability. Songs were seen to be central to the coping processes adopted within the therapeutic relationship in music therapy. Certainly, songs were a way for the individual to acknowledge mood states and implicit meanings whilst maintaining a coping front. Hence although an individual could sing about mood and emotional states which otherwise would be identified as 'not coping' or intolerable, within the music, such feelings were tolerated. It was only when verbal reflection took individuals too close to the issues at hand that coping strategies would be adopted, such as distracting or contradicting. This is a crucial issue for therapists who may be dismissive of an individual who expresses the wish to stay with the use of songs.

Consideration must be given to what the implicit meaning of the improvisations were for individuals, even when they could not articulate them verbally. Pavlicevic (1997) debates the primacy of 'meaning' versus 'creating'. The descriptions given by some of the participants in this study depict 'being' the music – that is, the music sounded as they were, defining their identities, through physical, emotional and interpersonal ways. However, the musical meaning remained allusive in their 'non-musician' interpretations. As chronically sick individuals, their interpretations revealed how much the music embodied their concepts of self. This may mirror what Pavlicevic describes as the 'portrayal of the client's experience of "himself-in-the-world" through sound'.

Individuals living with Multiple Sclerosis are desperate for a cure and this is central to their day-to-day existence. As music therapists, we have no cure to offer. Music therapists working with individuals with chronic incurable illness may well experience feelings of 'hopelessness' or 'futility' as they struggle to determine the focus of their intervention. As practitioners, we may be left with a feeling of 'there is nothing I can do'. Perhaps this offers another explanation as to why so little literature exists about music therapy and Multiple Sclerosis.

This is centrally important to the work with this client group. Without doubt, 'identity' is a central phenomenon in chronic incurable illness. The wider implications of this research are that as chronically ill individuals become weaker and more disabled, we are able to continue working with them, illuminating how music therapy may be able to address a central concept for every individual living with chronic incurable illness.

For these individuals, there are many factors which specifically affect the music therapy process. In mutual active music making, music therapy can be a highly physical experience for the chronically ill individual, in which they may monitor their own performance and way of being in the world. As therapists, we can validate our clients' performance through mutual music making, thereby facilitating a new concept of wholeness and aiding in identity reconstruction. In this way we can provide our clients with opportunities to challenge their illness identity. For those clients who are unable to physically manipulate instruments, or for whom the abstract nature of improvising is less meaningful, familiar songs which hold personal meaning can facilitate biographical work. Through their associative properties and the relationship held over time, songs operate on implicit and explicit emotional levels. Through the sensitive and therapeutic use of song, our clients can identify and experience emotional states which coping with their illness does not ordinarily allow.

Glossary

Ataxia: uncontrolled gross shaking movements caused by any intentional movement.

Grounded theory: a qualitative research method for analysis of data. The method categorizes data into conceptual units which are then grouped into subcategories and categories. Relationships between the categories are established by means of a paradigm which examines the properties of a

222 CLINICAL APPLICATIONS OF MUSIC THERAPY

phenomenon, the dimensions to these and intervening conditions which then impact upon interactional strategies.

Multiple-data sources: the use of more than one data source as part of the triangulation process.

Triangulation: a method used in qualitative research to increase validation by gaining interpretations from two or more perspectives.

Subcortical dementia: a term used to describe the cognitive changes seen in a number of neuro-disabling diseases such as Multiple Sclerosis, Huntington's Disease and Parkinson's Disease, characterized by the absence of aphasia, deficits in memory retrieval, impaired conceptual and reasoning skills, slowed information processing, personality disturbance, and characterized by depression or apathy. Other intellectual functioning may remain near normal.

Acknowledgements

I would like to acknowledge the supervision of Dr Jane Davidson in this research, the clinical supervision of John Woodcock RMTh, and the financial assistance of the Living Again Trust, the John Ellerman Foundation and the Juliette Alvin Music Therapy Fund. Most of all, I would like to thank those people who consented to be research participants in this study.

This work was undertaken by the Royal Hospital for Neuro-disability, which received a proportion of its funding from the NHS Executive. The views expressed in this chapter are mine and not necessarily those of the NHS Executive.

References

Aldridge, D. (1995) 'Spirituality, hope and music therapy in palliative Care.' *The Arts in Psychotherapy 22,* 2, 103–109.

Bailey, L. (1984) 'The use of songs in music therapy with cancer patients and their families.' *Music Therapy 4,* 1, 5–17.

Bright, R. (1986) *Grieving: A Handbook for Those Who Care.* St Louis: Magna Music Baton Music Inc.

Brooks, N. and Matson, R. (1987) 'Managing Multiple Sclerosis.' In J. Roth and P. Conrad (eds) *Research in the Sociology of Health Care: A Research Annual. The Experience and Management of Chronic Illness 6.* London: JAI Press Inc.

Butler, R. and Lewis, M. (1982) *Aging and Mental Health.* St Louis, MO: C.V. Mosby Co.

Charmaz, K. (1987) 'Struggling for a self: Identity levels of the chronically ill.' In J. Roth and P. Conrad (eds) *Research in the Sociology of Health Care: A Research Annual. The Experience and Management of Chronic Illness 6.* London: JAI Press Inc.

Conrad, P. (1987) 'The experience of illness: Recent and new directions.' In J. Roth and P. Conrad (eds) *Research in the Sociology of Health Care: A Research Annual. The Experience and Management of Chronic Illness 6.* London: JAI Press Inc.

Corbin, J. and Strauss, A. (1987) 'Accompaniments of chronic illness: changes in body, self, biography, and biographical time.' In J. Roth and P. Conrad (eds) *Research in the Sociology of Health Care: A Research Annual. The Experience and Management of Chronic Illness 6.* London: JAI Press Inc.

Lengdobler, H. and Kiessling, W.R. (1989) 'Gruppenmusiktherapie bei multipler Sklerose: Ein erster Erfahrungsbericht.' *Psychotherapie, Psychosomatik, Medizin und Psychologie 39,* 9–10, 369–373.

Magee, W. (1998) '*Singing My Life, Playing My Self. Investigating the Use of Familiar Pre-Composed Music and Unfamiliar Improvised Music in Clinical Music Therapy with Individuals with Chronic Neurological Illness.* Unpublished PhD thesis, University of Sheffield, England.

Mahler, M. and Benson, D.F. (1990) 'Cognitive dysfunction in Multiple Sclerosis: A subcortical dementia?' In S. Rao (ed.) *Neurobehavioural Aspects of Multiple Sclerosis.* Oxford: Oxford University Press.

Martin, J.A. (1991) 'Music therapy at the end of a life.' In K.E. Bruscia (ed.) *Case Studies in Music Therapy.* Philadelphia: Barcelona Publishers.

O'Callaghan, C. (1995) 'Songs written by palliative care patients in music therapy.' In C. Lee (ed.) *Lonely Waters: Proceedings of the International Conference on Music Therapy in Palliative Care.* Oxford: Sobell Publications.

O'Callaghan, C. (1996) 'Lyrical themes in songs written by palliative care patients.' *Journal of Music Therapy 33,* 2, 74–92.

O'Callaghan, C. and Brown, G. (1989) *Facilitating Communication with Brain Impaired Severely Ill People: Using Neuropsychology and Music Therapy.* Presented at N.A.L.A.G.'s Sixth Biennial Conference, Melbourne, September 1989.

O'Callaghan, C. and Turnbull, G. (1987) 'The application of a neuropsychological knowledge base in the use of music therapy with severely brain damaged adynamic Multiple Sclerosis patients.' *Australian Music Therapy Association Conference Proceedings,* 92–100, Melbourne.

O'Callaghan, C. and Turnbull, G. (1988) 'The application of a neuropsychological knowledge base in the use of music therapy with severely brain damaged disinhibited Multiple Sclerosis patients.' *Australian Music Therapy Association Conference Proceedings,* 84–89, Adelaide.

Pavlicevic, M. (1997) *Music Therapy in Context: Music, Meaning and Relationship.* London: Jessica Kingsley Publishers.

Rao, S. (1986) 'Neuropsychology of Multiple Sclerosis: A critical review.' *Journal of Clinical and Experimental Neuropsychology 8,* 5, 503–542.

Robinson, I. (1988) *Multiple Sclerosis.* London: Routledge.

Strauss, A. and Corbin, J. (1990) *Basics of Qualitative Research. Grounded Theory Procedures and Techniques.* London: Sage Publications.

Walton, J.N. (1977) *Brain's Diseases of the Nervous System, 8th Edn.* Oxford: Oxford University Press.

Whittal, J. (1991) 'Songs in palliative care: A spouse's last gift.' In K.E. Bruscia (ed.) *Case Studies in Music Therapy.* Philadelphia: Barcelona Publishers.

CHAPTER 12

Music Therapy in Neurosurgical Rehabilitation

Simon Gilbertson

Introduction

This chapter presents issues in the field of music therapy in neurosurgical rehabilitation and a general overview of the work being carried out in the Department of Music Therapy in the Klinik Holthausen.

The Klinik Holthausen

The Klinik Holthausen is a clinic for the early rehabilitation for patients who have been surgically or non-surgically treated following neurosurgical diagnostic procedures. The clinic was opened in January 1993 with a total of nine wards with 210 beds and expanded in January 1995 with two wards with 60 beds for the specialized treatment of children and adolescents. Between January 1993 and January 1999, 8180 patients have been treated in the clinic.

Patient profile in the Klinik Holthausen

The following section presents general information concerning the patient profile in the clinic. The largest proportion of patients admitted into the clinic have experienced some form of organic or morphological changes within the brain. This includes head injury or traumatic brain injury (TBI), intracerebral haemorrhage, cerebral aneurysm, tumour of the brain and cerebrovascular accident or stroke.

To gain an impression of the effects of such neurological illnesses, the occurrence of various functional disorders is shown in Figure 12.1. The information has been taken from a statistical analysis of patients treated in 1997 carried out by the Institut für Klinische Neurochirurgie in the clinic. The percentages do not total 100 as most patients do not present one single disorder but a complex of disorders.

These functional disorders include sensori-motor disorders, speech and language disorders, neuropsychological disorders (including disorders in spatial awareness and body awareness), constructive apraxia, and disturbance of consciousness and vegetative and coma states. Other common functional disorders include disturbance of micturition and intestinal function, shunt obligation and swallowing dysfunction. One of the most important factors concerning the success of neurosurgical intervention is the shortest time span between operation/trauma and the beginning of rehabilitation. The majority of the patients are admitted directly from intensive care treatment with an average time span of between two to four weeks between operation/trauma and admission to the Klinik Holthausen.

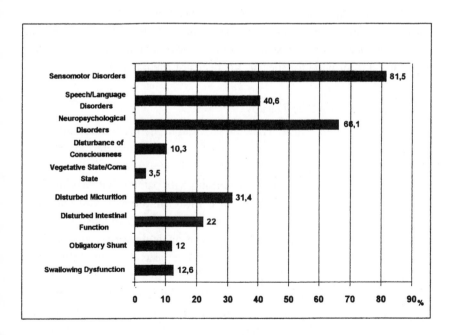

Figure 12.1 Functional disorders, admission 1997 (N = 1913)

Multi-disciplinary team

A multi-professional staff is essential to provide the best possible care and therapy for these patients. The staff in the Klinik Holthausen includes doctors (with experience in neurosurgery, neurology, psychiatry, internal medicine and paediatrics), nursing staff, physiotherapists, occupational therapists, balneological therapists, neuropsychologists, speech and language therapists, arts therapists and music therapists. At the present time there are seven music therapists working in the clinic in either full-time or part-time employment.

Since the opening of Klinik Holthausen in 1993, the development of music therapy has been possible due to the ongoing support from both the managing and medical directors during the realization and development of the clinic and also the process of 'growing up together' in a clinic which first opened six years ago. Similarly, the collaboration with the University Witten/Herdecke has played a significant role and will certainly continue to do so in the future.

The diverse groups of professionals working in the clinic have had the chance to learn where clinical boundaries have existed, where overlapping areas of clinical interest exist and where new overlapping areas have had to be adapted to provide for the specific needs of the patients.

The Department of Music Therapy

The Department of Music Therapy provides both individual and group therapy for up to 120 patients per week. Patients are referred to music therapy from all eleven wards. Over the past six years the music therapists in the clinic have gained experience in working with patients with a wide range of clinical symptoms. The diversity of clinical symptoms is vast and often specific within neurosurgical rehabilitation. The presence of music therapy in this field, in relation to other fields of application, is at a very early stage in its growth and many factors must be considered in the assessment of the overall development of the clinical application of music therapy in this setting.

The most significant factors to be considered include the level of training and education of music therapist after studies, the amount of experience therapists have had in other settings in order to develop associative thoughts on therapy and the infrastructure surrounding music therapy in the clinical institution. It is common that questions requiring the attention of researchers can develop out of observations made in clinical situations. An interaction between clinicians and researchers must be nurtured in order to gain from the combination of their activities and, as Aldridge (1996a) states, 'it is vital that we develop a sound basis of research-oriented clinical practitioners' (p.276). Thaut (1998) similarly suggests the need for an integrated system of practice and research and he accentuates that it should be based on music-related scientific research which could result in a widening of the music therapy profession. Within neurosurgical rehabilitation it is essential that clinicians have the opportunity to develop a scientific understanding of both music and medicine in order to be able to develop clinically relevant therapy interventions.

Music therapy

In general, the indications for music therapy within this field are not concretely defined and are continually being refined. This is due to the increasing experience of clinicians and the developing understanding of symptoms and disorders caused by neurological illness. Certain areas have grown in importance and interest during the past six years in the clinic (Weckel and Ischebeck 1995). These areas include work with patients affected by speech/language disorders, motor dysfunction, memory disorders, changes in personality due to organic damage, sensory disorders and changes in consciousness. Group therapy settings have been particularly developed for the treatment of the following groups: patients with changes in consciousness who present characteristics of vegetative states; patients with speech/language disorders; patients with organically caused changes in personality and one of its most severe forms 'Organic Brain Syndrome'; patients with disturbances of motor planning, motor co-ordination and muscle control; patients with difficulties in social relationships and integration as a direct result of brain trauma; and for children whose personal development and growth has been disturbed by brain damage and illness.

The following examples have been selected from the work of various music therapists in the clinic to highlight how interactive improvisation has been applied and understood during contrasting stages of treatment in early neurosurgical rehabilitation. Building upon clinical methods in improvisation learned in training, the therapists have been able to explore the appropriateness of this form of intervention with various groups of the patient population.

Clinical examples

Vignette 1

> Charlotte is a fourteen-year-old girl who was diagnosed within the para-
> meters of coma vigil as the result of a paraneoplastic limbic encephalus.
> Following admission to the Klinik Holthausen she presented a spastic
> tetraparesis, no spontaneous speech and no observable signs of
> awareness for her surroundings. The manner in which she perceives
> herself and her environment is impossible to define at this early stage.
> Whilst holding Charlotte's hand, the music therapist quietly begins
> singing short melodic phrases with small intervals which are repeated.
> Charlotte's staring eyes are motionless and directed away from the
> therapist. As Charlotte sighs deeply, the therapist's melody rises in pitch
> with larger intervals reflecting the change in her breathing. The text,
> 'hear your song', remains unchanged. Charlotte sighs deeply and the
> therapist lets go of her hand and she begins to turn her head slowly
> towards the direction of the therapist, who repeats the previous melodic
> phrase. A sense of the early signs of an intentional search for contact is
> felt by the therapist.

Moments such as these can assist developing speculation concerning the
patient's intentions and can be of use in the evaluation of the child's
responses to the therapist's actions – in this particular case improvised
singing. The use of repetitive melodic phrases can serve two purposes at this
stage: first, it can optimize the possibility of recognition for the listener and
the possibility to communicate this recognition to the therapist, and, second,
it is possible for the therapist to carefully use variations in dynamic, timbre,
tempo and structural form. This second element is of significance for the
therapist to be able to form a clarity of musical content and thus aid the
patient to form a 'catalogue' of parameter variables which is essential for the
development of a sense of expectancy and change. The singing voice is an
optimal communicative instrument due to its monophonic nature,
undisturbed by simultaneously occurring tones and complex harmonies,
which takes place within the natural physiological structure of breathing
patterns. This further increases the possibility of developing a basis of
understanding for the communicative interaction between patient and
therapist. This is a common process of development and is often used during
such early stages of therapy.

Changes within vegetative status begin with the first signs of communicative ability in the broadest sense of the word. This 'communicative ability'

can be observed in the form of motor activity following a request – for example, visual activity, eye contact or visual fixing – or reacting to the acoustic environment in the form of turning the head towards acoustic sources. Often, these observations can be categorized as forms of reflex, uncontrolled reactions and intentional reactions.

An important point to mention is that these early signs of communicative ability are not only specific to music or to music therapy. This fact is most seldom, if ever, mentioned within music therapy literature. These observations form an important basis of interaction within a wide range of situations – for example, during physiotherapy, nursing care and during contact between patient and family members. The most significant differences, at this stage, between music therapy interventions and the others lies in the relationship between humans and the medium of music itself and that the level of activity required for participation in an interactive activity (music) can be simplified and reduced to a minimum whilst retaining its essence. The therapist can base his/her improvisational activities, for example, on the breathing of the patient. In this context the patient can thus influence the course of the interaction through minimal changes in his/her breathing.

In the very early stages of music therapy with patients who are not physically stable enough to be mobilized in a wheelchair I have tentatively begun to look for alternative signs of change. One interesting area has been that of eye movement when the patient has either open or closed eyelids whilst I have been singing short improvised melodic phrases. Based on my studies of acoustic localization, I came across the topic of the 'audio-visual reflex' (Paulsen and Ewertsen 1966). This reflex is characterized by the moving of the eyes towards the source of perceived sound. Therefore, it was possible to hypothesize whether eye movement towards the direction of my singing could be interpreted as a sign of the development of active perception of my singing. Even when the patient has closed eyelids, through careful room lighting and a training of my awareness for such movement it was possible to chart the movement of the patient's eyes in relationship to the content of my singing. Once the initial localization reflex had taken place, I would then continue to sing until the eyes became restless and moved away from the 'site' of my voice. After a short pause the process would be repeated. Once a pattern between my singing and the patient's eye movement becomes recognizable, it is possible to hypothesize more definitely about the patient's awareness of his/her environment and surroundings. At this stage, this area of interest has been highlighted to aim at widening the manner in which the patient can be perceived and observed in a phase where changes in his/her life are often in minute dimensions.

Other minimal changes in the patients' activities, such as the movement of a limb or vocalization, can provide a platform for interactive activities. It is most important that the therapist makes most careful observations of changes so that patterns of change are maintained for possible communicative interaction. Gustorff (1990) reported in her work with patients in coma states where it was possible to search for, and to build up, contact through the singing of improvised melodies based on the musical elements (rhythm, intensity, dynamic) observed in the breathing of the patients. Weckel (1998), following this methodology, reports of his work with a patient suffering from apallic syndrome where he improvises vocally, concentrating on the breathing of the patient. He goes on to describe how the patient began to develop eye contact with the therapist during a music therapy session for the first time after half a year in the apallic syndrome. He states that the main role of music therapy in this situation can be described as 'the attempt to enter into contact' (p.41).

A clear differentiation should be made between the prognostic future for patients in coma and patients living in varying stages of vegetative state (see Glossary). The 'outcome' for patients is extremely diverse and the time span involved between observable change can range from days to years and, possibly, continue until death without any observable change. This differentiation must be made to ensure that the clinician develops adequate and suitable demands on the patient and does not develop false expectancies. The development of feelings of disappointment or of inadequacy in the therapist must be carefully worked through to avoid negative effects on the processes of therapy.

As previously mentioned, within improvisation the actions of the patient can be developed as intentional patterns of communication with the therapist. These patterns of musical communication are seen as a prototype for communicative patterns which possibly can be later transferred into other mediums of communication, such as gestures, 'codes for language' based on specific movements or averbal vocalizations. In the early stages, minute movements, changes in breathing or eye movement can be musically improvised upon and can provide communicative 'links' between patient and therapist and can function as a foundation for interaction.

Vignette 2

Michael is a nine-year-old boy who suffered severe brain injury in a car accident on 14 November 1996. Following neurosurgical treatment he was admitted into the Klinik Holthausen on 16 December 1996. At the time of admission he was diagnosed within the parameters of vegetative syndrome. It was not possible to enter into any form of interaction with him. He presented a right-sided tetraparesis and later developed hydrocephalus, whereby the implantation of a shunt was necessary. Early signs of brain atrophy were diagnosed following computer imaging.

One can, perhaps, imagine how such situations, as the result of a sudden, often devastating, event, can be riddled with challenging uncertainties, helplessness and hope for the future. The important moments in the early stages of Michael's music therapy were based on the observations made as he began to respond to the therapist. The therapist sings on a falling minor third interval to the word 'hallo'. Initially, Michael responds by gradually turning his eyes in her direction and begins to close and open his eyes. A short time later in the session the therapist interprets his opening and closing of his eyes as an offer to enter into a form of dialogue. It seems as though he changes the speed of his eye movement and begins to close and open his eyes in the tempo of her singing. A phrase is sung and the rhythmic continuum is carried forwards with an answer through the closing and opening of eyes. Built on simple processes such as alternation or the repetition of particular melodic patterns or changes in the accentuation of repeated melodies, a clarity in the organization of actions is maintained. Whereby the observation of Michael's eye movements is initially perceived as a response, following various repetitions it seems that this rhythmic closing and opening of eyes is an active impulse for the therapist to acknowledge this impulse with a repetition of the melody. This facilitates the evolution of an individual form of dialogue which is based on a mixture of musical (therapist) and non-musical (patient) communicative elements. Under careful observation, it is the child who adds the element of eye closing into the interaction and the therapists who reacts to this impulse. The resulting dialogue is complementary, balanced and unique to the individuals involved.

The discovery of such interactive possibilities within music therapy can lead to transfer outside of the music therapy setting. A common experience is that activities of dialogue, as mentioned previously, can lead to the development of a coded system of communication for basic and essential statements for use in everyday life. One example is the closing of the eyes and holding them closed for a moment to be interpreted as 'yes', and closing two times after another for 'no'. During the early phases of rehabilitation the application of relearned abilities in situations outside of the therapy setting, or between various therapeutical settings, demands well-informed interaction between members of the multi-disciplinary team. Often, it is the case that various therapists from contrasting areas concentrate on similar issues. These issues are co-ordinated between the team members and the optimal combination of therapy forms can aim at identified issues for concentration within therapy and provide a consistent and stable environment for the patient.

A group music therapy setting has been developed for adults who, in the early stages of rehabilitation, begin to show early signs of communicative ability. Minimal movement, early signs of meaningful eye contact and a questionable level of social awareness are the categories applied to define criteria for participation in this group. The choice of the term 'criteria' and not 'indication' is made to highlight the importance of the development of a flexible 'working model' in the clinical situation. This enables the development of therapeutic intervention based on the early observations of a wide range of patients presenting comparable levels of activity whereby the diversity of causality is large.

Vignette 3

Following a motorcycle accident causing cerebral contusion, skull and other skeletal fractures and severe acute complications, Mr G was admitted into the clinic in the middle of November 1997. Ten days after admission he began to receive individual music therapy and, one month later, began to participate in the aforementioned group.

In the initial phases of therapy the extreme reduction in the speed, dynamic and diversity of his movements determined the form of interaction. He physically presented a high level of muscle tone in his whole body, which caused his joints to be in either complete extension or almost complete flexion in a pattern of spasticity. Small arm movements, almost taking place in a time loop, were interpreted by the therapists as answers to questions concerning choice, participation and wishes. To maintain clarity it is important for the therapist, at this stage, to increase the level of consideration concerning which form of question and answer relationship exists and to assess the level of correct/false flexibility. Various verbal strategies can provide this required level of clarity, whereby questions based on expected yes/no answers can often offer the most reliability.

The first stages in therapy concentrated on forming an impression of his capabilities and limitations in being able to play various instruments which demanded a minimum of strength or complex co-ordination. It was necessary for a co-therapist to support his hand and arm movements as he presented a tremor-like movement pattern and extreme muscle weakness. Instruments such as a tambour, windchimes or lyre were offered in this initial phase to encourage 'facilitated impulses' in the production of single tones and sounds.

As time continued, the therapists continued to aim at facilitating the exploration of new possibilities based on the patient's existing motor skills. The concept of using music in therapy concentrating on increasing motor skills has existed for a relatively long period (Fields 1954) and provided new thoughts for consideration in therapy. Alternation between facilitated beating on a drum and a reduced level of physical intervention from the therapist allowed Mr G to re-experience movements and to explore his own physical capabilities. Melodies based on simple binary rhythms played on the piano were used to support and connect single tones which he produced on percussion instruments and provided him with a structured temporal continuum for the organization of his movements. The sounds which he created were interpreted by the therapist in terms of basic musical elements, rhythmic, tonal and dynamic. Improvised accompaniment offered the optimal chance to both accompany the speed of his actions and to reflect the quality of his playing. This form of expressive reflection in interactive improvisation cannot be defined with any one particular formula. Often, qualities such as physical tone can be reflected in harmonic tension. Harmonic patterns develop during the course of improvisations and remain flexible in variational changes between tension and relaxation.

During the further course of rehabilitation Mr G developed more and more communicative ability and personal identity in various situations in the clinic. At this stage, music therapy played the role of providing 'free improvising interaction' – most of the other therapies concentrating on rigidly determined aims such as developing first steps into non-pathological walking patterns or exercises in dressing and undressing himself. He also began an intensive stage of self-reflection and adaptation to his personal situation in life. Whilst regaining cognitive skills and an increase in awareness of his physical and psychological new 'self', he gained more insight into the restrictions and handicaps which remained issues of considerable uncertainty. Through the well-known context of improvisation, the bridge towards increasing self-dependency and responsibility for the course of the improvisations existed. Similarly, the group setting provided him with an opportunity to enjoy and develop relationships with other patients during group improvisations where each member was encouraged to play without externally defined rules or extensive instruction from the therapists. Support was offered where requested and words and gestures of encouragement were exchanged between all members. The chance to continually explore possibilities and limitations within a setting characterized by 'doing' music, with the possibilities of creative freedom, was of great importance at this stage in his overall personal development. This also provided him with an opportunity simply 'to be' (Aldridge 1996b) in a phase of his life characterized by remaining 'deficits' and demands from others 'to become'.

The role of active music therapy with patients affected by speech/ language disorders concentrates on the development of interpersonal musical activity and the development of emotional expression.

Various factors have played a role in the developing interest and understanding of the relationship between music and speech, particularly in the fields of neurological research, speech rehabilitation and musical expression. The following section portrays how developments in these fields have influenced the understanding of the role which music therapy can play in the early rehabilitation of patients affected by aphasia.

Aphasia is the term used to describe 'a disturbance of the comprehension and formulation of language caused by dysfunction in specific brain regions' (Damasio 1992). All aspects of speech and language can be affected – the disturbance of speech production, understanding of the spoken word, understanding of the written word and the combinations of these elements. Since 1861, as the neurologist Pierre Paul Broca discovered a patient who could understand the spoken word but who had no speech production (Kandel, Schwartz and Jessel 1995), the search for the site in the brain (localization) responsible for specific behaviour has continued to play an important role in the study of the brain. Interestingly, this very first report of such a patient included the further description that the patient 'could utter isolated words and sing a melody without difficulty but could not speak grammatically or in full sentences, nor could he express ideas in writing' (p.12). The examination of the brain, following the patient's death, revealed damage to the left hemisphere posterior to the frontal lobe. This phenomenon of a seeming discrepancy between the ability to sing and not to speak has continued to be an issue for discussion up to the present day. One hundred and twenty-seven years have passed and uncertainties continue to remain in the understanding of this phenomenon. Studies, which included the intracarotid injection of sodium amylobarbitone which inactivates one hemisphere of the brain, perhaps highlight the extent researchers have gone to in trying to solve this matter (Gordon and Bogen 1974). Perhaps the human strive towards 'understanding' has maintained the level of presence of this issue in continuing related studies. The developments in modern technology, such as magnetic resonance imaging and computer-based tomography, have sharpened the argumentative evidence for the specification of the localization of human behaviour. Studies during the past ten years have been characterized by brain images taken from 'normal subjects' whilst performing strictly controlled tests with the aim of defining these 'responsible areas' through measurements of changes in cerebral blood flow and metabolic processes (Sergent et al. 1992). This information aids the development of essential scientific understanding of human behaviour and can be then added to the development of clinical therapy strategies. Often, reference is made to studies of music and functional neuroanatomy and the function of music in patients affected by aphasia caused by left hemispherical damage (Alajounanine 1948; Gates and Bradshaw 1977; Keith and Aronson 1975; Sparks, Helm and Albert 1974). However, relatively few examples of the development of models for music therapy strategies based on such information appear (Lucia 1987). The formulation of therapeutic interventions based on these findings must be further expanded. Similarly, a differentiation between the aims of these various interventions could assist during the selection of appropriate modalities of treatment for music therapists working in the clinical setting.

The following statements present a selection of the main considerations surrounding issues in music therapy: whether 'musical expression' can offer a meaningful alternative for verbal expression; whether the similarities between speech and music in human activity provide enough substantial evidence for the formulation of models of therapy based on the 'musical' elements found in speech; whether localization theories of speech and music in the brain can shed light on the discussion of how these two seemingly similar activities could be related; whether it is possible to order the descriptions of phenomena experienced with patients affected by aphasia , such as the ability to 'sing' words which cannot be spoken (Morgan and Tilluckdharry 1982) and whether the historical course of interest/studies has really lead us to an appropriate manner of reflection and speculation. I suggest that the non-localized or non-exclusive hemispherical localization for musical activity must be seen as a key concept in the furthering of our understanding of this scenario. Clinical experience has shown that patients affected by such severe speech/language disorders often maintain the ability to enter into musical improvisation with another person. In the therapeutical setting, using active improvisation, it has been a primary aim at developing and realizing the individual potential for musical expression within a relationship based on interactive music making. The aim of applying this form of intervention is not simply to rehabilitate speech but to operate as a part of the multi-disciplinary rehabilitative intervention process. Music therapy concentrates here, in the early stages of developing an interactive situation, on aiming at increasing the patient's intentional entering into interpersonal situations in and outside of the music therapy setting.

Other developments not involved with active improvisation concentrating on the work with patients with aphasia are mentioned later, in the section 'Other areas of clinical importance for the future'.

Vignette 4

Following subarachnoid haemorrhage and intracerebral haemorrhage, Mr D experienced a disturbance in all modalities of speech and language (global aphasia), which prohibited verbal communication, and began to develop early signs of social isolation. He showed no signs of physical dysfunction. Up to the time of illness, Mr D was a proficient hobby musician and enjoyed playing classical music on the piano. His individual music therapy was characterized by instrumental improvisation. In one particular session, through the use of pointing, he chose a set of five woodblocks from a selection of melodic and percussive instruments to play with the therapist at the piano. Out of the stillness of reflection he began to carefully try out the five tones of the woodblocks. During this initial phase he only looked down at his instrument whilst playing. Each tone was repeated once or twice and then he moved to the next tone. By imitating the quiet, short staccato nature of his playing and the number of times each note was struck, the therapist reflected his playing in her playing at the piano. After a short time, perhaps half a minute, he looked up from the woodblocks, entered into eye contact with the therapist and grinned. He had, perhaps, recognized the intention behind the music coming from the therapist and recognized a relationship between his playing and the therapist's playing. Suddenly, the two players became almost simultaneously louder and faster and a sense of rhythmic organization for the exchange of rhythmic patterns developed. The improvisation continued with exchanges of rhythmic motives, mood qualities and a wide range of stylistic forms which both players could recognize and respond to. Verbal interaction was not possible due to the total involvement of both players in music making and, during this activity, was not a hindering element in interaction.

Mr D's initiative towards self-expression through music and the modulation of expressive qualities in his playing enabled the development of a relationship with the therapist. He could enter into musical interaction with another person, which was not possible in verbal communication. It is a valid hypothesis that the areas of his brain needed for music production and perception were fully intact and not directly handicapped by the damage to the left hemisphere which caused severe disturbance of his speech and language ability. Therefore, the use of music as a therapeutic medium aimed at not only encouraging interactive experience within the music therapy setting but also at providing Mr D with positive experiences, increasing his confidence to enter into other communicative situations in daily life and within other forms of therapy.

Vignette 5

Being affected by Wernicke's aphasia and a right-sided paresis, Mr K's ability to understand the spoken word and the production of comprehensible speech was severely reduced. In a conversation with his brother it became clear that Mr K had been involved with music since his childhood and during his adult life had conducted a children's choir and was a proficient musician. The damage to his brain extended into the pre-motor cortex, the area included in movement planning and co-ordination. He found it almost impossible to beat in a steady pulse, not able to control the direction of the beater and improvisations were characterized by arhythmic, almost chaotic, beating in an uncontrolled and uncoordinated manner. It was necessary to assess whether, or to what extent, his musical comprehension and motor ability could be affected. In such situations the therapist must develop the ability to differentiate clinical observations in order to be able to make informed decisions concerning subsequent forms of therapeutic intervention. It was to put to question whether physical uncoordination or cognitive understanding of music itself could be causing his difficulties in making music. Later in therapy it was possible for Mr K to retrain physical co-ordination and control in time and space when facilitated by a clear musical content and structure. The temporal organization of the movements he needed to beat were supported through the temporal organization and accentuation of the music played by the therapist. The content and structure was often based on steady binary rhythms, with a constant harmonic tempo – for example, chord changes taking place every four bars and a harmonic language based on chord patterns such as I, IV, V. This form of the organization of movement in a music-based temporal structure supported Mr K in the development of physical co-ordination and, furthermore, increased his ability to emotionally express himself in instrumental improvisation with the therapist.

It has become obvious during the past years that musical expression cannot provide a substitute for verbal expression. However, the ability to enter into musical interaction in improvisation can offer the expression of emotionality, an opportunity to be heard and listened to, and, most significantly in early stages of rehabilitation, raise the level of personal value – which can lead to a reduction of avoidance of entering into any form of communication and contact with others.

Developments for the future

For the greater number of patients suffering from a subarachnoid haemorrhage of the anterior communicating artery, the development of neuropsychological and psychopathological symptoms is most common. Various grades of severity in cognitive disturbances are observed in the areas of memory, concentration, problem solving, attention and cognitive flexibility. Changes in personality, thought processing, affection and drive are also observed. The most severe grades of Organic Brain Syndrome present extreme disturbance in orientation to all qualities, elements of paranoid tendencies and the false recognition of people and places, with the possible tendency to run away. The Klinik Holthausen has pioneered the development of a facultative half-closed ward providing for the specific needs of this patient group. Music therapy is offered in both individual and group settings. Early observations are beginning to form specific considerations concerning possible adaptations of therapeutic intervention.

One example of these activities is concerned with the development of the group therapy setting for patients being treated on the facultative half-closed ward.

It is being considered that, due to severe disorientation in time, the significance of the basic temporal structure in music may increase to such an extent that almost all initial group improvisations are characterized by a monotonous tempo and reduced rhythmic variation. Furthermore, the impression is gained that, without further intervention, the group would continue playing without pauses or phrasing for an extended period of time. Interventions concentrating on raising the participants' ability to organize temporal structure within music may be of help in providing a model of temporal and structural organization which can be transferred into daily life. The use of group improvisation also aims at facilitating an increase in orientation to person and place. The representation of musical activity within memory processing could provide a trigger to the formation of recall and recognition information. Naturally, due to the pioneering nature of this work, more time is needed to gain experience and for the development of specific therapeutic strategies based on the individual needs of patients living with Organic Brain Syndrome.

Other areas of clinical importance for the future: 'Clinical Neuromusicology'

The role of music therapy in the Klinik Holthausen has been portrayed here through a presentation of a small fraction of its application which has concentrated on aspects of active improvisation and musical interaction. There are, however, other areas of clinical interest and importance for future development. To adapt and move away from concepts and methodologies learned during therapy training can be experienced as an intricate and, sometimes, insecure process. I feel, however, that the future development of music therapy in early rehabilitation following neurosurgical treatment must look towards a widening of its applications. This widening of applications could include an adaptation of already existing applications and methods taken from other clinical settings – for example, receptive music therapy, guided imagery in music or analytic music therapy – or be based on the development of new applications developed specifically for neurosurgical rehabilitation. Many of these present developments are at early stages – the following examples aim to highlight the areas of interest developed in the

Klinik Holthausen, and is not an extensive discussion of the continually changing issues within these areas.

Following a visit to learn of the work by Thaut in the Center for Biomedical Research in Music, Colorado State University, USA, and an examination of the literature (Davies 1995; Lucia 1987; Thaut 1985), studies have begun to assess whether music-based motor rehabilitation could be adapted and integrated into the Klinik Holthausen. A study of the effects of music-based intervention based on physical rhythmic synchronization to music and acoustic feedback of movement whilst relearning to walk, with patients presenting hemiparesis whilst receiving treatment from physiotherapists on the treadmill, has increased interest for future interdisciplinary collaboration.

A music-based test is being devised to identify and document disturbance of basic musical function in patients presenting aphasic symptoms. In fourteen steps of graduated difficulty, the test aims to measure the patients' perception of musical events through the analysis of their musical reproduction of these events. It concentrates on two fundamental musical concepts: the division of a time continuum and its compound form, rhythm and melody. Simple percussion instruments, such as snare drums, are used for the rhythmic steps and the singing voice for the melodic steps of the test. Similarities and differences between what the therapist and patient have played or sung are documented to analyse whether patterns of difference become apparent. Computer-based amplitude analysis of digital audiotape recordings made during the test is used to support the aural findings of the therapist and to provide the possibility for objective data analysis. Through studying the morphological condition of the brain with the use of Magnetic Resonance Imaging and incorporating other forms of information (for example, EEG results), it has been possible to begin to compare specific musical phenomena and disorders of music perception and production within the context of neurological damage causing aphasic disorders.

A pilot study has been carried out to investigate the effects of three-dimensional hearing activities during the rehabilitation of a patient with hemi-neglect and hemi-anopsia following traumatic brain injury. Patients suffering from lesions or trauma of the non-dominant posterior parietal lobe (usually right) often show an agnosia, a perceptual neglect of the left side of the body, disturbing the body image and their perception of spatial awareness. Based on theories of spatial hearing (Blauert 1974), designs were made for a three-dimensional acoustic framework using up to ten loudspeakers at various points around the listener. It was hypothesized that the ability to discriminate the origins of acoustic events can provide the patient with an alternative spectrum of information concerning his/her environment, thus increasing the perception of spatial awareness (Blauert 1983). Using information gained from the acoustic environment, it is expected that the patient can also significantly develop motor ability – including an increased body awareness, hand–eye co-ordination and an increased recognition of stimuli within their surrounding space. The single tone and music signals to be used were selected in conjunction with research carried out into tone recognition (Blauert and Lindemann 1986, 1985; Boucher and Bryden 1997; Wiens, Emmerich and Katkin 1997). The hypothetical expectations made pre-trial were confirmed during the study and the patients' spatial awareness of the contra-lesional hemi-space increased to such an extent that the percentage values for correct answering during +90 degrees to -90 degrees acoustic awareness tests increased from 51 per cent at the outset of the study to 92 per cent in the final stage of the study. Further diagnostic and treatment interventions are being considered based on the findings of this pilot study. Acoustic localization therapy interventions are being further developed for patients affected by visual disturbances, such as post-trauma blindness, or for patients following severe damage or removal of one eye. Such disturbances are relatively common for patients following head injury and this form of intervention has begun to play an important role in the treatment of patients in rehabilitation following neurosurgery. Such activities as these also provide extra information which can be put to use within other modalities of therapy. Information gained in acoustic perception and spatial hearing can be integrated into active improvisation settings where it can be made possible for patients to begin to take part in group improvisation activities – for example, through the identification of the spatial relationships between the various group members a significant increase in the comprehension of the acoustic environment can be developed.

Contemporary developments within neurology, neurosurgery, neurophysiology and neuropsychology have led to a widening of interdisciplinary interest in other professions. The study of the human brain with modern technology has begun to include more and more studies of the role of the brain during musical activity (Barret 1995; Sergent et al. 1992).

The term 'Neuromusicology' has been used in conjunction with studies concerning the relationship between the brain and music. A limited usage of the term 'Neuromusicology' is to be found in the literature (Hart 1998). However, a growing number of studies in this field are taking place and in June 1997 the congress 'The Foundations of Neuromusicology' held in the University of Gent accentuated the increasing interest in this new field. The development of the clinical application of findings in 'Neuromusicology' presents the need for a new perspective in the definition of direction in clinical music therapy. In April 1998, at the 4th European Congress for Music Therapy, I stated the importance and significance of neuromusicology in the furthering of clinical music therapy in early rehabilitation following neurosurgery. The development of a new field, 'Clinical Neuromusicology', is suggested here to fulfil this need and to be defined as: the scientific and clinically applied branch of neuromusicology concerned with the study, diagnosis and treatment of patients living with brain damage/illness.

Particularly in the area of rehabilitation following neurosurgical intervention, the clinical adaptation of neuromusicological findings can begin to take place. Innovative diagnostic and therapeutic strategies can be developed based on the findings of modern research. I believe that the two elements of 'time' and 'harmony' in the relationship between clinicians and researchers could lead to a symbiosis of ability and understanding which will surely play an important role in the future development of neuromusicology and clinical neuromusicology.

Summary

This chapter has presented the context of music therapy in neurosurgical rehabilitation and the various roles music therapy has played for patients treated in the Klinik Holthausen. Considerations concerning active music therapy in this specific field, with various patients and possible areas for future development, have also been mentioned. The integration of neuromusicology has been highlighted and I have suggested that clinical neuromusicology could provide a defined and appropriate field for growth for the application of music in therapy for patients affected by neurological illness. The chapter has been aimed at increasing interest in this most fascinating and challenging area, where the application of music therapy is called upon to continually develop and realize theoretical potential into therapeutical reality.

Glossary

Aphasia: a category of language disorders resulting from a lesion to specific structures in the brain. These include: Broca's aphasia, Wernicke's aphasia, conduction aphasia, paraphasia (Kandel, Schwartz and Jessel 1995).

Central nervous system (CNS): one of the two anatomical divisions of the nervous system, the other being the peripheral nervous system (PNS). The central nervous system comprises of the brain and spinal cord. Although anatomically separate, the central and peripheral nervous systems are interconnected functionally (Kandel, Schwartz and Jessel 1995).

Cerebral contusion: a form of brain damage caused by extreme movement of the brain – often caused by a blunt impact to the skull which results in diffuse multiple haemorrhages and damage on the opposite side of the brain (Contre-Coup). Most commonly affected are the frontal-basal and temporal-basal regions.

Clinical neuromusicology: scientific and clinically applied branch of neuromusicology concerned with the study, diagnosis and treatment of patients with brain damage/illness.

Entrainment: a term used to describe the process of rhythmical motor synchronization to a rhythmic acoustic source.

Neglect syndrome: a syndrome associated with lesions of the posterior parietal cortex, manifested by a neglect of the opposite side of the body (Kandel, Schwartz and Jessel 1995).

Neuromusicology: field concerning the scientific study of relationships between the brain and music.

Vegetative state: a clinical condition of unawareness of self and environment in which the patient breathes spontaneously, has stable circulation and shows cycles of eye closure and eye opening which may simulate sleep and waking. This may be a transient stage in the recovery from coma or it may persist until death (Bates 1996).

References

Alajouanine, Th. (1948) 'Aphasia and artistic realization.' *Brain 71*, 3, 229–241.

Aldridge, D. (1996a) *Music Therapy Research and Practice in Medicine: From Out of the Silence.* London: Jessica Kingsley Publishers.

Aldridge, D. (1996b) 'The body, its politics, posture and poetics.' *The Arts in Psychotherapy 23*, 2, 105–112.

Barret, J. (1995) 'The quest to map the brain: Manhattan project of the mind.' *The Mission 22*, 1, 4–14.

Bates, D. (1996) *The Vegetative State: Continuing, Persisting, Permanent?* Proceedings taken from Joint Conference of the British Medical Association, King's College Centre of Medical Law and Ethics and the Office of the Official Solicitor, London.

Blauert, J. (1974) *Raeumliches Hoeren.* Stuttgart: S. Hirzel Verlag.

Blauert, J. (1983) *Spatial Hearing – The Psychophysics of Human Sound Localisation.* Cambridge, MA: MIT.

Blauert, J. and Lindemann, W. (1985) 'Spatial mapping of intracranial auditory events for various degrees of interaural coherence.' *Journal of Acoustical Society of America 79*, 3, 806–813.

Blauert, J. and Lindemann, W. (1986) 'Auditory spaciousness: Some further psychoacoustic analyses.' *Journal of Acoustical Society of America 80*, 2, 533–542.

Boucher R. and Bryden, M.P. (1997) 'Laterality effects in the processing of melody and timbre.' *Neuropsychologia 35*, 11, 1467–1473.

Davies, P.M. (1995) *Wieder Aufstehen: Frühbehandlung und Rehabilitation für Patienten mit schweren Hirnschädigungen.* Berlin: Springer Verlag.

Damasio, A.R. (1992) 'Aphasia.' *The New England Journal of Medicine 326*, 8, 531–539.

Fields, B. (1954) 'Music as an adjunct in the treatment of brain-damaged patients.' *American Journal of Physical Medicine 33*, 273–283.

Gates, A. and Bradshaw, J. (1977) 'The role of the cerebral hemispheres in music.' *Brain and Language 4*, 403–431.

Gordon, H.W. and Bogen, J.E. (1974) 'Hemispheric lateralization of singing after intracarotid sodium amorbarbitone.' *Journal of Neurology, Neurosurgery and Psychiatry 37*, 727–738.

Gustorff, D. (1990) 'Lieder ohne Worte.' *Musiktherapeutische Umschau 11*, 120–126.

Hart, S. (1998) *Overtures to a New Discipline: Neuromusicology.* http://www.columbia.edu/ci/21stC/issue-1.4/mbmmusic.html

Kandel, E.R., Schwartz, J.H. and Jessel, T.M. (1995) *Essentials of Neural Science and Behaviour.* New Jersey: Prentice Hall Publishers.

Keith, R.L. and Aronson, A.E. (1975). 'Singing as therapy for apraxia of speech and aphasia: Report of a case.' *Brain and Language 2*, 483–488.

Lucia, C.M. (1987) 'Towards developing a model of music therapy intervention in the rehabilitation of head trauma patients.' *Music Therapy Perspectives 4*, 34–39.

Morgan, O. and Tilluckdharry, R. (1982) 'Presentation of singing function in severe aphasia.' *West Indian Medical Journal 31*, 159–161.

Paulsen, J. and Ewertsen, H.W. (1966) 'Audio-visual reflex: Determination of the audio-visual reflex in directional hearing by employment of electronystagmography.' *Acta Otolryng. Supplement 224*, 211–217.

Sergent, J., Zuck, E., Terriah, S. and MacDonald, B. (1992) 'Distributed neural network underlying musical sight-reading and keyboard performance.' *Science 257*, 106–109.

Sparks, R., Helm, N. and Albert, M. (1974) 'Aphasia rehabilitation resulting from Melodic Intonation Therapy.' *Cortex 10*, 303–316.

Thaut, M.H. (1985) 'The use of auditory rhythm and rhythmic speech to aid temporal muscular control in children with gross motor dysfunction.' *Journal of Music Therapy 22*, 3, 108–128.

Thaut, M.H. (1998) 'Wer und was fordert die Musiktherapie in der Zukunft? Wissenschafts-theoretische Grundlagen, Forschungsmodelle und therapeutische Anwendungen.' *Musiktherapeutische Umschau 19*, 1, 15–20.

Weckel, J.W. (1998) 'Musiktherapie in der neurologischen Rehabilitation. Apallisches und Post-komatöses Syndrom.' In D. Aldridge (ed) *Kairos II: Beitrage zur Musiktherapie in der Medizin.* Bern: Hans Huber Verlag.

Weckel, J.W. and Ischebeck, W. (1995) 'The importance of music therapy as a modality in the treatment of patients with cerebral lesions.' *Book of Abstracts, 3rd European Music Therapy Conference, 81.* Aalborg, Denmark: Aalborg University Press.

Wiens, S., Emmerich, D.S. and Katkin, E.S. (1997) 'Response bias effects perceptual asymmetry scores and performance measures on a dichotic listening task.' *Neuropsychologia 35*, 11, 1475–1482.

PART FOUR

Aspects of Training
and Clinical Supervision

CHAPTER 13

Integrative Supervision for Music Therapists

Isabelle Frohne-Hagemann

Roots

Integrative approaches to supervision for music therapists are based on the concept of 'Integrative Therapy' that integrates different 'schools' of therapy with psychoanalytical humanistic, social scientifical and artistic backgrounds. Some psychoanalysts that have had influence are, for example, Sandor Ferenczi (1931), who offered the concept of parenting, reparenting and mutuality; Wilhelm Reich (1949), who introduced body work into therapy; Otto Rank (1975), who realized very early on the necessity of developing creativity and creative self-realization; Michael Balint (1988), who emphasized the aspect of interpersonal relationship; and Vladimir Iljine (1942), who developed the therapeutical theatre. Gestalttherapists of importance were Fritz Perls, R.F. Hofferline and Paul Goodman (1951) and the inventor of psychodrama, Jakob L. Moreno (1946). From the side of philosophy, Integrative Therapy was much influenced by existential philosophers like Gabriel Marcel (1969), Jean Paul Sartre (1962), Maurice Merleau-Ponty (1966), and by phenomenological philosophers like Martin Heidegger (1957), Hans-Georg Gadamer (1978), and Hermann Schmitz (1964–1981) as well as by social-constructivists like Paul Watzlawick (1977), Thomas Luckmann (1979) and Niklas Luhmann (1971).

Integrative Therapy was developed by Hilarion Petzold in the 1960s (Petzold and Sieper 1993). This concept is taught in several study programmes with different therapeutic accents at the 'European Academy of Psychosocial Health' (Fritz Perls Institute for Integrative Therapy, Gestalt therapy and Promotion of Creativity). I met Petzold in 1977 and was trained in Integrative Gestalt psychotherapy and movement therapy at the institute. As a music therapist with, at that time, a more pedagogical background, I here found basic therapeutic concepts that convinced me and gave a frame for what I wanted to do in music therapy. The broad range of creative and person-oriented interventions, of different approaches to healing modalities, the training concepts with an accentuation of self-experience and 'learning by doing', as well as the concepts for supervision, confirmed and enriched my own ideas.

Integrative Music Therapy

On the one hand, 'Integrative Music Therapy' (IMT) can be regarded as a method of 'Integrative Therapy' (IT) because of the same basic philosophical, sociological, ethical, anthropological and therapeutical roots. On the other hand, IMT offers concepts that, in their turn, enrich Integrative Therapy and characterize IMT as a self-reliant method. Music philosophers like Victor Zuckerkandl (1963, 1964), pedagogues like Heinrich Jacoby (1983) and music therapists of different 'schools' like Helen Bonny (Bonny and Savary 1973), Mary Priestley (1975), Christoph Schwabe (Schwabe and Röhrborn 1996), and many others, have influenced IMT.

The term 'integration' should not be misunderstood: it is a principle, not a 'school'. Integration does not mean to use a little bit of this and a little bit of that and mix it together in an unreflected way. Integration means to be interested in a 'culture of coping with variety' (Petzold 1997) in order to do justice to the plurality of ways of living and understanding. Integration means to seek connections and transitions between different theoretical and practical conceptions. As human beings do not perceive the world with only one sense but with at least five senses, it seems logical to take in 'polyphonic' perspectives in order to find adequate approaches to our clients and supervisees. Clients in different situations and with different diseases and symptoms need different therapeutic approaches. Many perspectives have to be integrated and, as Fritz Perls once said, 'There is no end to integration.'

Supervision as an integrative concept

One of the subjects taught in our training course is supervision. With regard to supervision, integration is based on the confrontation with the theories and praxeologies with which music therapists work. In a supervision group with supervisees from different backgrounds it is most exciting to explore the plurality of theories and praxeologies for compatibility.

Supervision for music therapists gives an impression of our integrative concepts and I will explain some of them in this chapter. I will put the emphasis on hermeneutics and a model of supervision that integrates different music therapy theories and techniques. For many years music therapists and supervisors all over the world have created very interesting and effective music therapy techniques from different basic philosophies. In a hermeneutic model these techniques can be used to make clear the different ways of understanding and handling therapeutic situations. The examples I will give later, however, will, of course, not present a complete classification of music supervisional techniques.

In order to explain the foundation of this model, I will first make a rough draft of the basic positions of IMT.

Some metatheories of IMT

IMT takes in an ecological viewpoint and follows the Heraklitian wisdom of 'panta rhei'. Everything is connected with everything and in constant motion. Reality is never final and creation is a never-ending process. It is not only creation but co-creation (Petzold 1990) because creation is the result of relationship and exchange. Thus man is a co-creator of genesis and responsible for mankind's future. Music therapy, as a creative method, can help our clients to take an active part again in our genesis. IMT is a creative and, therefore, process-oriented therapy.

Co-creation needs 'co-respondence' (Petzold and Sieper 1993), which is also one of our central concepts. To *respond* implies a relationship. *Co-respond-ence* is a 'rhythmical' (Frohne 1981) way of reciprocal interacting and communicating. Being in 'resonance' (Frohne-Hagemann 1990; Petzold, 1980, 1993c) is, to me, more than being in 'respondence'. It is an active and consciously experienced perception of the relationship between 'the other' and one's self and can be regarded as an emotional attunement within the interaction (German: *Ko-Respondenz*). If individuals are in musical interaction and also resonating to the common musical gestalt they are part of, the result can be a sharing of realities. This leads to the construction of a third reality, a consensus that contains the different social worlds of individuals. Emotional attunement and exchange, however, takes place at different levels of maturity and ranges in many variations of interaction, such as between a confluence and inter-subjective encounter. Music therapy has as an aim the establishment of a musical relationship that allows therapy partners to differentiate the levels, widen the fixed forms of relationships and experiment with empathy, response and resonance.

This concept has influence on our valuation of health and disease. Because of the process orientation, the diagnosis of a client's health or disease can, viewed anthropologically and ecologically, only be formulated as a hypothesis because diagnosis has to take into consideration the reciprocal relationship of client and therapist and the contemporary spirit of the scientific, cultural and daily age in which they live.

Perception is always *intentional* (Husserl 1948), which means that as perceiving and acting persons we are always intentionally relating to the world. What we hear, see, touch, smell and taste is dependent on our intentions, convictions, beliefs and so on. These are influenced and affected by our cultural, social, historical and political 'lived worlds' (Husserl 1962) and these change through the years and centuries. There is an inter-determinism in that, in the span of our perception, we decide what will be perceived (Hensel 1980). It is very important to be aware of this because it helps us to be careful with 'the truth' of one theory and careful with interpretations that could stigmatize a client. In IMT not only our therapeutical focus but all metatheoretical assumptions are process oriented and need constant discourse. The supervisional model I will present later should also be understood as a hypothesis in a process which only becomes useful if it finds consensus.

The anthropology of the creative person

The German term *'Leib-Subjekt'* (Petzold 1984) is a very complex concept that cannot comprehensively be translated into English. The best translation would be the 'person in the world'. We are a composition of body, soul and mind (spirit) in an insoluble relation to our milieu and our history. The *'Leib-Subjekt'* is an ecological concept. The person in the world is a sociological, psychological, physiological person in the dimensions of space and time. The development of our identity takes place by processes of interaction, starting in the mother's womb with reciprocal stimulation and continuing with emotional and social attunement, social interaction and processes of finding consensus in the perception and understanding of different social realities. The identity of the *'Leib-Subjekt'*, the 'person in the world', is not stable. There is no definite core self or 'true self' but a vulnerable identity constantly striving after balance and coherence. The creative person is like the musical self, a flowing energy striving after form and gestalt (which is 'identity'). As in music, this development demands repetitions thousands of times in order to construct an identity, a stable reality. Music is like the flow of the musical self finding different ways (coping strategies) of forming a musical gestalt (personal and social identity) with the help of its musical ego. Experiments (in improvisations), experiences and many repetitions of emotionally meaningful experiences are necessary in order to develop the capacity of memory and a reliable reality (object relation). We can observe this in music therapy as well when we may accompany our clients' development of their expressive and formative musical competence in relation to the development of their identity. If a person can live musically (related, expressive, changeable and yet structured), he or she can be called healthy in a deeper sense. This also means that he or she is cultivated.

Music is important to experience the process of constructing a coherent identity by 'living' the time, and music therapy is an indispensable method to enable such a cultivation, especially for clients who missed adequate stimulation in the sensitive phases of their development. A cultivated person with a coherent identity has differentiated and refined his or her abilities of perception, of memory and of both verbal and non-verbal forms of expression. The cultivated person is able to construct a reality that makes sense, that gives him or her identity when times and conditions change, a reality or world that can be shared , modified or changed with others. His or her reality is not fixed, it is recreated and co-created with others every single day. A cultivated person is a healthy person, which means that he or she has the possibility to grow. He or she is flexible and adaptable to changes, as in music.

This is the main statement of our 'anthropology of the creative person' (Frohne-Hagemann 1990; Petzold and Orth 1988). This anthropology believes that knowledge develops in the form of a creative spiral – perception, memory, expression in their dialectical relationship with cognition and the analogous and digital modes of reflexivity. The creative, healthy person is not dependent on one 'single vision' attitude as he or she has the ability to look at phenomena from different perspectives. He or she can take in a dualistic, external viewpoint (for example when he, as a surgeon, has to cut into a body and thus has to regard a person as a piece of flesh) but he or she is not fixed to that.

Paths of healing

These are, presented briefly, the main global aims of IMT. How do we achieve them? In regard to therapeutic consequences our anthropology takes two aspects into consideration: treatment of *clinical diseases*, such as depression, early disturbances, etc., and treatment of *sociological diseases*, such as alienation. These two directions implicate different paths of healing: music therapy as a psychotherapeutic treatment (paths 1 and 2) and music therapy as promotion of creativity and development of solidarity and cultural and political engagement (paths 3 and 4). To be the healthy (cultivated) person is the goal of all paths of healing and education and, of course, these four paths can only be separated from each other by a theoretical perspective. In practice they complement each other:

Psychotherapy:

- The search for meaning in one's life, insight in damaging narratives, liberation from fixed ideas and emotions. It is a path where, for example, suppressed feelings and conflicts are uncovered and solved. Mostly, we are involved in treating neurotic clients.

- The development of basic faith and self-confidence, a path of reparenting and experiencing healthy relationships in order to make up for deficit experiences, to give support, to try to repair disturbed structures and to cope with traumatic experiences. This path is for early damages that have their origin in a time before the baby could express itself verbally. It is also called the sovereign art of psychotherapy.

Agogics:

- The development of potentials, resources and creativity by self-experience. This path is one for normal persons as well for those who want to broaden their horizons.

- The development of solidarity, cultural engagement and metaperspectives with regard to social and political processes of alienation. This path focuses on anthropological values on a therapeutic level.

(See Petzold 1993d; Frohne-Hagemann 1990, 1996)

IMT, therefore, takes into consideration the great etiological plurality of sorrow and handicap, and uses music therapy approaches that range from unstructured improvisations and the stimulation of fantasies with music (in order to free the unconscious material) to pedagogically and developmentally oriented modes of intervention (in order to stimulate and direct certain developments). The music therapist can be a facilitator, a screen for projections, a teacher/educator, a counsellor and much more. At all levels he is a resonator who is a part of the therapeutic process.

Epistemology

In our approach to understand (musical) realities we use the phenomenological and hermeneutic method. The reality of any experience has its own subjective truth. Music cannot be 'interpreted' without problems. But with the help of the phenomenological method we can try to 'reconstruct' a person's actions, motivations, decisions, etc. This can be done in different ways. I want to mention just two of them.

Reality and subjectivity can be reconstructed in a dialectical interaction between the phenomena and our pre-knowledge (prejudice) about the phenomena and structures of their reality. This method was developed by Gadamer (1978), a student of Heidegger. As Petzold (1993b) formulated further, the hermeneutic process proceeds in a spiral from the perception of the phenomena to a point where we seize the connections and meanings of the event/scene in a pre-verbal holistic way. From there the spiral takes its course to the phase where we emotionally and intellectually understand what is going on and find words to describe it. The last phase we reach would be the phase of explanation where we are able to explain the experience from different perspectives and levels. If we cannot explain (interpret), we have not yet understood. This spiral is never-ending. Each explanation or interpretation is the starting point for new perceptions and what we have explained will influence everything we will perceive in future. This again is a reason to work in a process-oriented way of diagnosis – which means that we constantly build hypotheses and do not rigidly classify what a client has. I have formulated this method for IMT in order to understand a musical expression or interaction (Frohne-Hagemann 1990b).

Within this process the reconstruction (and also a new construction) of the client's reality will also be built up by empathy and identification with him and with parts of him, such as his feelings, his behaviour, his psychological age, his dreams, etc. This method is derived from a romantic tradition that Dilthey (1957) had introduced. The technique of identification was developed further in gestalt therapy and is also used in IMT, as I will show later. As mentioned earlier, in IMT we work with the concept of 'resonances'. As a therapeutic 'technique' in music therapy, this concept leads to a greater understanding of transference and countertransference. Resonance is a way to interact with each other's reality, to let oneself be emotionally touched and to share emotions to a degree that is supporting the client.

Research into linguistic rules that represent general mechanisms of communication and actions are of great interest within IMT as we understand music as a linguistic code based on common action and inter-subjective communication in social contexts, which includes emotional qualities. Music is like the mother tongue, it does not not just stand for the English or German language but for a competence that enables us to feel the meaning of a word or an expression in its context (Frohne-Hagemann 1991). This is a very corporal phenomenon. In my opinion, music can only be felt in co-respondence to our basic corporality. In a way, the 'Leib-Subjekt' feels musically. We feel the qualities of emotions by breathing with the music, we 'taste' the meanings of musical gestures corporally. Perception, seizure and understanding are often connected with musical qualities such as atmospheres, feelings and rhythmical structures that illustrate a scene. Daniel Stern's (1990) musical description of Joey's experiences is a good example. Joey *perceives* the world musically and he is *seized* by the (musically experienced) atmospheres of the outside world and he can only later organize (rhythmically) the phenomena to something meaningful (which is *understanding*). However, he cannot yet *explain*.

Now, what do all these epistemological assumptions mean for supervision?

Supervision

First, let me make some general statements. If a music therapist has had a training as a supervisor, he or she functions as a counsellor, not as a therapist. This means that the supervisor looks at the personal problems of the supervisee only in so far as they interfere with his actual work with his client or his team. Thus the supervisor is not a therapist of the supervisee and his work is not primarily focused on people's personal problems.

Supervision, in my opinion, covers two wide areas: counsel – supervision of therapeutic relationships and cases (including training) – and treatment of actual conflicts at one's place of employment.

In the following I will describe the areas of supervision with regard to group supervision and individual supervision. Both can be combined as it is possible that a supervisee works on a problem with the help of the supervision group.

Counselling

CASE SUPERVISION (SUPERVISION OF THERAPEUTIC RELATIONSHIPS)

In my model the focus lies in the relationship of the client and the supervisee, on transference and countertransference, on the uncovering of blocks and repressed or unconscious material the supervisee and his/her client suffer from within the therapeutic process. The understanding of the musical relationship between the client and his/her therapist is, in this context, special and demands specific interpretation.

CASE DISCUSSION

The focus to work lies in the 'case'. The client's anamnesis, diagnosis, his/her background, his/her emotional and social development, the understanding of the client's musical expression, the adequacy of the therapeutic aims and methods, techniques and interventions, including the adequacy of the setting, timing, agreements, etc. Of course, the development of a case can only be understood as a figure in front of the therapeutic relation.

SUPERVISION AS CONTINUOUS TRAINING OF THERAPISTS

The focus lies on the supervisee's personal, social and professional competence and performance (including musical skills) – that is, his/her ability for empathy and authentic response, his/her awareness for transference, countertransference and resonance, also on the reflection of the supervisee's political, cultural, philosophical background, his/her diagnostic conceptions, his/her use of clinical concepts, methods and techniques, his/her competence and performance of working in different settings and with different clients and their different environments, etc.

Psychotherapeutic research (Petzold and Sieper 1993) has found out which unspecific values have therapeutical influence. Without them, no specific music therapy intervention would be efficient. Therefore, a supervisor should create among the supervisees of a supervision group a warm accepting atmosphere which allows them to learn and improve their abilities by personally experiencing and living the values they regard to be therapeutically important. The values are in this order: empathy, emotional support, practical help, promotion of emotional expression, promotion of experiences of evidence, meaning and insight, promotion of being well-connected, promotion of awareness and psychophysiological relaxation, promotion of learning processes and interests, promotion of creative experiences and formation, planning of the future, promotion of positive personal values, promotion of a clear feeling of one's own identity, promotion of social networks, experience of solidarity.

Thus empathy and emotional support are the most important values a music therapist should be able to present. It should be self-evident that these three categories of counselling cannot be exactly separated from each other in practice.

The treatment of actual conflicts at one's place of employment

- Team supervision: the focus lies in the understanding, facilitating and enabling of communication and co-operation with and among colleagues, nurses, superiors, holding organizations, etc.

- Organization: the focus lies in giving advice in case of changing a job, position, on handling negotiations, etc.

- Clinical management: the focus lies in giving support to lead a ward for music therapy or to set up a practice for oneself.

Although the second area is a field that has great influence on the actual therapeutic work of a music therapist, I would like to restrict myself in this chapter mainly to the first area. My hermeneutic heuristic is supposed to help supervisees to understand, explain and improve their music therapy work.

This model could also serve as a heuristic for research reasons because each phase needs considerable time to process. During a normal group supervision of two hours it will not be possible to follow the model in the perfect way. The model is a heuristic which allows shortcuts and skips as it becomes necessary.

The spiral (Figure 13.1) takes into consideration the aspects of hermeneutics as well as selected therapeutical working through and training. Therefore, it looks a little different from the hermeneutical spiral mentioned earlier (perceiving, seizing, understanding, explaining).

Each of the four phases of the spiral discuss a certain focus on the presented problem in supervision, which can be tackled with the help of music therapy techniques that approach the problem either from a

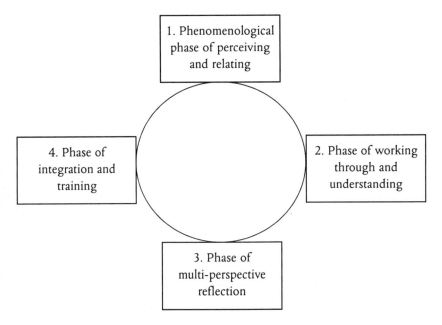

Figure 13.1 An integrative model for supervision of music therapy situations

psychoanalytical, humanistic or other perspective. Different music therapy methods and techniques thus correspond to these phases in a specific way.

The phenomenological phase of perceiving and relating

The themes found in this beginning phase include: What is the topic? What does the supervisee report about the 'figure' in front of the therapy process, the group relationships (if he or she leads the group in music therapy), the psychodynamic aspects, the actual context, the therapeutic situation? What and how do we as supervisors and group members perceive? How does the supervisee's report effect us and how do we resonate to that?

Useful improvisations in this phase are, for example: the 'Music therapy Balint-group improvisation' (Loos, Strobel and Timmermann 1988); the 'Empathic countertransference' (Priestley 1997b); the 'Spontaneous amplifying improvisation'(Weymann 1996); and hermeneutic techniques such as 'Analysis of tapes' (Weymann 1996), 'Criteria for the hermeneutic of music therapeutic processes and improvisations' (Frohne-Hagemann 1991, 1997). These are techniques we often use in the field of counselling.

The music therapy Balint-group improvisation / empathetic countertransference

Both are based on a psychoanalytical approach and work with the phenomena of transference/countertransference.

Example: the supervisee, Peter, has verbally introduced a problem he has with a patient in his hospital. Peter feels that the patient, a woman aged 28, plays 'games' with him. She does not want to improvise and is resistant to all of his suggestions. He feels angry and would like to become strict and hard towards her. At this moment, the members of the supervision group will play out their countertransference, which will help give Peter new insights about his patient. The group improvisation shows the polarity of anxiety on the patient's side and the provoked strictness on the therapist's side, which illuminates the basic role configuration of the patient and, perhaps, her father as well as her transference and resistance towards Peter. If he hears his feelings of countertransference, the strict behaviour, mirrored in correspondence to the patient's anxiety, he can get more information about her emotional world. For the group, this technique is also a very good training in basic therapeutic competencies such as empathy and response.

The spontaneous amplifying group improvisation

Weymann (1996) describes this technique as a spontaneous group improvisation that occurs right after the verbal introduction a supervisee has given to the group members. Weymann considers this technique to be very helpful when a verbal introduction only touches the surface of the problem (for example, if the problem concerns an early traumatic experience, or if the report arouses feelings that have to be repressed by the listeners, or if the group is too tired and a psychological change of perspective could be helpful). The technique reminds me a little of Freud's free-floating attention, but it can also be regarded as a music therapy technique where the 'music person' (in analogy to Nordoff/Robbins's 'music child') relates to the world in a tuned way. It is a wonderful way to feel yourself into the therapeutic situation and relationship of the supervisee and his client(s). This technique, in my opinion, leaves space for both working with one's feelings of countertransference and including one's own personal resonance. Two important aspects come into the discussion: countertransference as a reaction to empathy ('I feel how you feel or how your father felt, etc.') and resonance as an authentic answer to the relationship ('I offer you my own feelings to what you are and what you do'). This discrimination can be useful for case supervision and case discussion.

Let us assume that the group had played a spontaneous improvisation after Peter's report. There are many feelings – those of countertransference and resonance. It is very interesting to experience how the therapeutic process is repeated in the process of listening. After the improvisation, the first step into the hermeneutic spiral will be the ingenuous and spontaneous gathering of impressions and associations to the 'object' music.

In regard to the phenomenal approach to the music, the setting, the report of the supervisee, etc., the following criteria could help give an idea of what to be aware of. These criteria were actually developed for the use in therapeutic situations (Frohne-Hagemann 1991, 1997). What does the music therapist have to be aware of after he or she has improvised with the client or after the group has improvised? This model, however, can also be useful in supervision because the improvisations of the supervision group can more or less mirror the 'real' (original) therapeutic situation and its context. The list of criteria does not claim to be complete. Peter and the members of his supervision group will gather impressions and notice phenomena as listed in Figure 13.2.

According to the first column of the criteria, the members of the supervision group and Peter will be aware of atmospheres, emotions, feelings, body sensations, actions, fantasies, scenes, metaphorical thoughts, imagery, associations, memories, narrations. These should be verbalized in order to find hypothetical assumptions and consensus regarding the themes Peter's patient brings in. Peter might find out that his patient arouses associations like 'one does not dare to breathe', 'lost in a black hole', 'if you meet her you turn into a monster', and so on. What seems to become obvious in this case is the patient's feeling of being a victim. In order to support or modify or change this hypothesis the perceptions should be differentiated as much as possible with respect to the musical phenomena, the rapport, the relational levels and patterns, the choice and function of instruments, the behaviour and social function, the responses and resonances, transferences and countertransference, and so on. Peter might find, in columns 2–10, many hints from the music (even if the music is not an original tape of an improvisation with his patient). For example, the music could reveal 'flowing and stagnating' (column 2), 'overstimulations' (column 6), 'avoiding', 'feigning to be in contact' (column 7), and so on.

1. General impressions	Atmospheres, emotions, feelings, body sensations, actions, fantasies, scenes, metaphorical thoughts, imagery, associations, memories Narrations (what does the music tell us?)
2. Musical phenomena	Connections by pulse and rhythm; spectrum of sound, melody, phrase, variation, dynamic, texture, form; timing, intervals Response to the interaction of corporality and music: to become wider and narrower, flowing and stagnating, holding fast and letting go, breaking out and holding back, adapting oneself and resisting, etc.
3. Playing behaviour, personal expression	Corporal expression, muscle tension, colour of face, co-ordination of hands, head – hands, eye contact, mimic, gesture, attitude, approach to the instrument, etc.
4. Choice, function, coping with instruments	Carrier of symbols, area of projection, transitional object, intermediary object
5. Level of relationship	Isolation, confluence, contact, encounter, bond (negative: commitment)
6. Forms of contact (interventions and stimulations): too much, too little, adequate	Supporting, holding, framing, protecting, calming, reinforcing, confronting, provoking, listening, forming, varying, changing, etc. reciprocal homogene stimulation (adequacy?), inconstant stimulation (disturbances?), contradictory stimulation (conflicts?), overstimulation (traumata?), understimulation (deficits?)
7. Pathological and saluto-genetical forms of contact	Avoiding, breaking off, burning one's boats, blurring, dissolving, pretending to be dead, (anaesthesia), blocking, boycotting, splitting, becoming silent, playing with oneself, melting into one another, attacking, drowning a sound, sticking obstinately to something, harmonizing in any situation, playing perfectly, answering inadequately, feigning to be in contact, imitating, playing funny, playing in a give and take mode, archaic contact (immature), neurotic and mature forms

Figure 13.2 Criteria for the hermeneutic of music therapy processes and improvisations

8. Transference and counter-transference, resonance	Concordant, complementary, reciprocal, projective identification Mirror twin Role configurations such as mother and baby, strict father and naughty son, etc.
9. Role configuration in a therapy group	Alpha or Omega-type, harmonist, the grumbler, the scapegoat, the director, the watcher, the actionman, the judge, the angel, the 'therapist', etc.
10. Pre-knowledge	Concerning the client's identity: body, social net, work, material resources, values; concerning the familiar, social, political, cultural background; concerning the 'Musical life panorama' (MLP) and biography

Figure 13.2 Criteria for the hermeneutic of music therapy processes and improvisations (continued)

The next step in this phase would be to find consensus about the different perceptions, feelings, assumptions and conceptions that have been gathered by the group members. In Peter's case the consensus might be the hypothesis that his patient was abused and, therefore, cannot trust her therapist.

This first phase will give us much information in a rather wide sense. We are very much in the 'here and now' and busy with perceiving, feeling and relating. The next phase is the phase of working through and understanding, where we have a closer look at the problems Peter, our music therapist, has to cope with. This phase has therapeutic aspects – we trace the problem back to its roots and into its context.

The phase of working through and understanding

The themes found in this phase include: What does the obvious cover? Where does the therapist know this problem from? What is the emotional background or structure? What is the underlying emotional context and/or underlying picture that always leads to mechanisms of mutual transference/countertransference? What are the strategies the supervisee and his or her client develop in order to construct their reality? Where are the blocks and resistances of the client and of his or her therapist?

Useful improvisations are: 'The Musical Portrait'(described by Weymann 1996), 'Identification' and 'Symbolic Musical Interview'(Frohne 1986), 'Music Therapy Role Plays', and others.

The musical portrait

In this approach Peter would be asked to paint a musical portrait of his patient and to choose the adequate instruments. He chooses the quite tiny kalimba and plays it in a rather destructive way. This portrait is regarded as a mirror of the relationship the therapist feels towards his client and (in his opinion) vice versa. Thus the portrait reveals his own projections. It seems the patient has to be punished, but she also was punished and punishes herself.

The therapeutic attitude of the supervisional approach is quite different from the Balint work. The focus here lies much more on the problems the therapist has with the client, and the group members look at therapeutic situations as intermediate encounters.

In this case Peter is confronted with his own impulses to punish the victim and he begins to ask himself whether he cannot bear the feeling of becoming helpless himself. At this moment he is much more in contact with his inner resonances to the basic problem both partners share than with his feelings of countertransference. I believe this is the meaningful moment for a change in therapy. Peter might start to share his feeling of helplessness with his traumatized patient and this will help both to continue the therapeutic process.

If the supervision takes place as supervision within a team, another colleague could paint a musical portrait of Peter's patient and both improvisations would then be compared by members of the supervision group. This technique, in my opinion, is very helpful in the supervision of a therapeutic relationship because it tells more about the supervisees' feelings of countertransference, transference and resonances.

Music therapeutic identification

This is a psychodramatic and gestalt therapy approach with a systemic and social constructivist perspective. This technique in supervision is applied as a musical portrait from the projected client's view. The supervisee, Peter, identifies with his patient and directs a musical reconstruction of her situation. He can tell the members of the supervision group to play certain emotional qualities and social roles for him – for example, the emotional climate at home or the role of his patient's father or the role of himself as the therapist. The very consciously directed improvisation puts the focus on the patient's point of view and how the therapist assumes the client is experiencing him. Peter chooses two instruments for his patient: a drum and a stringed instrument. He plays in a hard and longing way and distributes both instruments to group members. He composes, with the help of the others and some instruments, an atmosphere of anxiety and listens to the music in identification with his patient. By doing so he imagines himself as the therapist who is asking his patient to improvise with him. Now he feels how threatening and seducing this must be for her and he understands how, unwittingly, he is put into the role of the aggressor.

This technique, together with the musical portrait, is very useful for case supervision and case discussion. A great amount of empathy is necessary for both techniques. It serves also for training issues. A variation of the identification technique (and maybe easier for some people) is the following.

The supervisor could ask the supervisee to be his or her client, to identify with an instrument and/or a musical motive that stands for that client, and interview him: 'What kind of drum are you? What is your nature? What do you need? How and under what conditions do you sound sane? How would you like people to play for you? What will you give them in return?' While answering, the supervisee might play the chosen instrument or just touch it, and answer musically and verbally at the same time in order to get a better flow of thinking and feeling.

Music therapy techniques like these are techniques that help one get a feel for adequate feelings, behaviours and interventions in respect of the client. Working through the emotional involvement means to find out about one's own transferences to the client and to see the connections of the problem in relation to the client. A warm sharing in the group is important for the emotional climate. A music therapist is very sensitive and needs support in his anxiety to fail. It is hard for Peter to feel his anxiety and anger towards his patient and the incapability to cope with his helplessness.

In order to find out what are the most efficient methods and techniques to reach the client in his coping with his personal and social conflicts, disturbances and deficits, there should be time to reflect, classify and arrange the insights and experiences in a multi-perspective way. This would help make better use of one's creativity and to try out new and different music therapy approaches.

Phase of multi-perspective reflection

The theme here is the understanding of the experiences from different perspectives. There are (at least) four dimensions that have to be considered if integration should make sense (Petzold 1996). Peter will have to answer to the following dimensions.

The political dimension

Where is the balance of power? What are the politics of the government? What is the actual situation of the public health service, traditions, cultures of institutions? Who pays and who is paid how much? We cannot be good supervisors if we do not consider the political, social and cultural conditions in which a music therapist has to work. For example, does Peter have the support from his team to treat a traumatized patient with music psycho-therapy? Will he lose his job if he does not function in the expected way? Where does he stand in the hierarchy? Does he have a full-time job at the hospital or is he working part-time?

The theoretical dimension

What are the 'philosophies' of the music therapist, his concepts of cognition, knowledge and diagnosis, his concepts of personality, of psychological development, of health and illness, his concepts of therapy, in general, and of music and, especially, music therapy, and his theories of music therapy methods and processes? What would Peter answer here?

The group will contribute to a great variety of perspectives. If a member of the supervision group comments on a therapeutic theme from a systemic perspective by pointing out a client's role as a scapegoat in his therapy group, or if another one comments on the topic from the psychoanalytical perspective of his countertransference, and if a third one comments on his feeling of not being in contact with the scene (a gestalt therapy perspective), the supervisor will point out the backgrounds of these therapeutic perspectives and concepts and will try to find transitions. Different music therapy methods and techniques with different theoretic backgrounds – such as psychoanalytical and social science positions – can complement each other and widen our horizon. If our theoretical background becomes broader and richer, we will also become more competent in staying open for different ways of understanding. From what perspectives can the theme Peter brought in be discussed?

The practical dimension

What professional background does the music therapist come from? What are the orientations of the field he works in? Maybe Peter has a gestalt therapy background but works in a hospital with psychoanalytic orientation. What does this mean with regard to the music therapy he offers to abused patients?

The respective ethical position

This concerns basic attitudes such as the decision for a focus on a relational premise or on linear or discoursive thinking. This is a very important dimension and has great influence on everything we do in therapy.

As a result of these experienced and reflected approaches, the phase of integration and training will follow.

Phase of integration and training

The themes found in this phase include: What are the consequences for the clients? How could the problems be solved by the supervisee? How can we improve our therapeutic skills?

Useful improvisations should be experimental, in order to find and test out more efficient musical approaches to, and musical interventions for, the client. Useful techniques could be music therapy experiments with inter-therapy (Priestley 1997b), role playing, verbal approaches, etc.

Inter-therapy/role plays

This method here can very well be used for the continuous training of therapists. The supervisee (or a student) will choose a group member to take the role of the therapist, whereas he or she will play the role of his/her client or vice versa. Different music therapy approaches will be practiced by going into the situation. It is always exciting to experiment with difficult situations. Peter, for example, will play his patient and different members of his supervision group will try to reach him verbally (as she did not want to touch the instruments) and musically, if possible. Different situations can be 'simulated' in the supervision group (where they often very quickly turn out to become 'real') and the different possibilities to intervene musically and verbally can be experienced and discussed from the different therapeutical attitudes. Peter might have to find out that he (in her role) needs more time and that it would be helpful if he, as her therapist, would just be present and patient.

The training effect, in my opinion, is not a result of using recipes but of being in contact (interaction and resonance) with the 'client'. From here creativity is born and the right channels to the clients will be found organically. (Of course, certain *musical* skills still might need some practising.) The group functions as a supervisor and will give emotional sharing and professional feedbacks to the 'therapist' and the 'client'. Inter-therapy can also be used for group therapy. In this case the main supervisor supervises the whole process from an external position.

Verbal training

How does the music therapist communicate? How does he enter into a conversation and dialogue and how does he bring a subject to the point? How does he deepen and work through the process after the musical improvisation and how does he lead the client into the phase of reflection and integration? What words and sentences does he use and how does he use them in difficult situations? How do the different psychoanalytical, systemical, gestalt therapeutic and other courses of conversation influence the music therapist?

In this phase of integration and training the focus lies very much on the aspect of the utilization of experiences and insights. All music therapists in the supervision group profit from the colloquial understanding as it influences their way of perceiving and relating to new problems. But, as I said before, the end of the spiral is always the beginning of a new one and there is no end to integration of the different worlds we live in and there will never be an end to learning from our colleagues, supervisees and our clients.

Glossary

Case discussion: a field of supervision where the focus lies on the client, his/her disease, social and psychological development, his/her actual context and situation, and so on. Discussed will be the adequacy of music therapy methods and techniques, not the problems of the therapist or his relationship with the client. A case discussion takes place when the supervisee and his/her supervisor discuss questions such as: What do we have to be aware of if we work with borderliners (psychosomatic patients)?

Case supervision: a field of supervision where the relationship between client and music therapist are focused upon. A musical improvisation dyadic or group situation can only be understood with the help of case supervision because the therapist is as much part of the client's reality as vice versa. Supervision mostly starts from case supervision in order to find solutions for the final case discussion.

'Leib-Subjekt': German term by Hilarion Petzold for the entity of body-self, psyche, mind and milieu. The 'Leib-Subject' is creating its identity in the span of life starting from an archaic body-self and archaic ego functions and developing, in interaction with the world, a rather coherent identity by integrating identifications of the world and those from the world.

The music therapy Balint-group improvisation: Use of Michael Balint's concepts in music therapy, especially in order to work with phenomena like countertransference.

Spontaneous amplifying improvisation: term used by Weymann. The Jungian term 'amplification' is a method to work with dreams. Weymann uses it for musical improvisation.

References

Balint, M. (1988) 'Changing therapeutical aims and techniques in psychoanalysis.' *International Journal of Psychoanalysis* 31, 117–124.

Bonny, H. and Savary, L. (1973) *Music and Your Mind: Listening with a New Consciousness.* New York, Evanston, San Francisco, London: Harper & Row.

Dilthey, W. (1957) *Die Entstehung der Hermeneutik, Gesammelte Schriften.* Göttingen, Stuttgart: Vandenhoeck & Ruprecht.

Ferenczi, S. (1931) 'Kinderanalysen mit Erwachsenen.' Bausteine III, 490–510. In Schriften III 274–289.

Frohne, I. (1981) *Das Rhythmische Prinzip, Grundlagen, Formen und Realisationsbeispiele in Therapie und Pädagogik.* Lilienthal: Eres.

Frohne, I. (1986) 'Musiktherapie auf der Grundlage der Integrativen Gestalttherapie.' *Musiktherapeutische Umschau* 7, 2, 111–123.

Frohne-Hagemann, I. (ed) (1990) *Musik und Gestalt. Klinische Musiktherapie als Integrative Psychotherapie.* Paderborn: Junfermann. Reprinted in 1999: Göttingen, Vandenhoeck and Ruprecht.

Frohne-Hagemann, I. (1991) *Musiktherapeutische Diagnostik und Hermeneutik.* Unpublished paper used at the music therapy study programme at the 'European Academy of Psychosocial Health' (Fritz Perls Institute).

Gadamer, H.G. and Boehm, G. (1978) *Seminar: Die Hermeneutik und die Wissenschaften.* Frankfurt: Suhrkamp.

Heidegger, M. (1957) *Identität und Differenz.* Pfullingen: Neske.

270   CLINICAL APPLICATIONS OF MUSIC THERAPY

Hensel, H. (1980) 'Die Sinneswahrnehmung des Menschen.' *Musiktherapeutische Umschau 1*, 3, 203–218.

Husserl, E. (1948) *Erfahrung und Urteil.* Hamburg.

Husserl, E. (1962) *Phänomenaologische Psychologie.* Hesserliana, Bd. IX, µ. Nijhoff, Den Haag.

Iljine, V. (1942) *Das therapeutische Theater.* Paris: Sobor (russ.).

Jacoby, H. (1983) *Jenseits von Begabt und Unbegabt.* Hamburg: Hans Christians Verlag.

Loos, G., Strobel, W. and Timmermann, T. (1988) 'Die musiktherapeutische Balintgruppenarbeit.' *Musikther. Umschau 9*, 4.

Luckmann, T. (1979) 'Persönliche Identität, soziale Rolle und Rollendistanz. In O., Marquard and K. Stierle (eds) *Identität.* München: Fink.

Luhmann, N. (1971) *Soziologische Aufklärung. Aufsätze zur Theorie sozialer Systeme.* Opladen: Westdeutscher Verlag.

Marcel. G. (1969) *Dialog und Erfahrung.* Frankfurt: Knecht.

Merleau-Ponty, M. (1966) *Phänomenologie der Wahrnehmung.* Berlin: de Gruyter.

Moreno, J.L. (1946) *Psychodrama.* Volume 1. London: Beacon House.

Perls, F., Hefferline, R.F. and Goodman, P. (1951) *Gestalt Therapy.* New York: Julian Press.

Petzold, H.G. (1980) *Die Rolle des Therapeuten und die therapeutische Beziehung.* Paderborn: Junfermann.

Petzold, H.G. (1984) 'Vorüberlegungen und Konzepte zu einer integrativen Persönlichkeitstheorie.' *Integrative Therapie 1*, 2, 73–115.

Petzold, H.G. (1990) 'Form und Metamorphose als Fundierende Konzepte für die Integrative Therapie mit Kreativen Medien – wege Intermedialer Kunstpsychotherapie.' In H.G. Petzold and I. Orth (eds) *Die neuen Kreativitätstherapien.* Paderborn: Junfermann.

Petzold, H.G. (1993a) 'Integrative Therapie. Modelle, Theorien und Methoden für eine schulenübergreifende Psychotherapie.' *Reihe Integrative Therapie. Schriften zu Theorie, Methodik und Praxis, 3 volumes.* Paderborn: Junfermann.

Petzold, H.G. (1993b) 'Der "Tree of Science" als metahermeneutische Folie für Theorie und Praxis der Integrativen Therapie.' In H.G. Petzold. *Integrative Therapie. Modelle, Theorien und Methoden für eine schulenübergreifende Psychotherapie, Volume II/2.* Paderborn: Junfermann.

Petzold, H.G. (1993c) 'Integrative fokale Kurzzeittherapie (IFK) und Fokaldiagnostik – Prinzipien, Methoden, Techniken.' In H.G. Petzold and J. Sieper (eds) *Integration und Kreation,* Volume 1. Paderborn: Junfermann.

Petzold, H.G. (1993d) 'Integrative therapie in der Lebensspanne.' In H.G. Petzold *Integrative Therapie. Schriften zu Theorie, Methodix und Praxis, vol. II/2*

Petzold, H.G. (1996) 'Materialien zur Integrativen Supervision und Organisationsentwicklung – "Supervisiorische Kultur", "Reflexives Management", "Konflux".' *Europäische Akademie für psychosoziale Gesudheit (EAG).*

Petzold, H.G. (1997) 'Supervisorische Kultur und Transversalität-Grundkonzepte Integrativer Supervision.' *Integrative Therapie 1*, 2, 17–59.

Petzold, H.G. and Orth, I. (1988) 'Metamorphosen -zur Arbeit mit kreativen Medien in der Integrativen Therapie.' In H.G. Petzold and I. Orth (eds.) *Die neuen Kreativitätstherapien.* Paderborn: Junfermann.

Petzold, H.G. and Sieper, J. (eds) (1993) *Integration und Kreation*. *Modelle und Konzepte der Integrativen Therapie, Agogik und Arbeit mit kreativen Medien*. Jubiläumsband, Volume 1. Paderborn: Junfermann.

Priestley, M. (1975) *Music Therapy in Action*. London: Constable and Company Ltd.

Priestley, M. (1997a) 'Musiktherapeutische Erfahrungen. Grundlagen und Praxis.' Stuttgart, New York, Kassel, Basel, London: Bärenreiter Verlag.

Priestley, M.(1997b) 'Erste Erfahrungen mit Intertherapie. Betrachtungen über den Klienten im Therapeuten und seinen Supervisor.' *Musikther. Umschau 17*, 3, 4.

Rank, O. (1975) *Art and artist*. New York: Agathon Press.

Reich, W. (1949) *Character Analysis'* New York: Orgone Institute Press.

Sartre, J.P. (1962) *Das Sein und das Nichts. Versuch einer phänomenologischen Ontologie* Reinbek: Rowohlt.

Schmitz, H. (1964–1981) *System der Philosophie*. 10 volumes. Bonn: Bouvier.

Schwabe, Chr. Röhrborn, H. (1996) *Regulative Musiktherapie. Entwicklung, Stand und Perspektiven in der psychotherapeutischen Medizin*. Stuttgart: G. Fischer.

Stern, D. (1990) *Diary of a Baby* New York: Basic Books.

Watzlawick, P. (1977) *Die Möglichkeit des Andersseins*. Bern: Huber.

Weymann, E. (1996) 'Supervision in der Musiktherapie.' *Musikther. Umschau 17*, 3, 4.

Zuckerkandl, V. (1963) *Die Wirklichkeit der Musik. Der musikalische Begriff der Außenwelt*. Zürich: Rhein Verlag.

Zuckerkandl, V. (1964) *Vom musikalischen Denken*. Zürich: Rhein Verlag.

CHAPTER 14

Psychoanalytically Oriented Music Therapy Supervision

Janice Dvorkin

The concept of supervision as part of the training of a psychotherapist was initiated in the psychoanalytic training institutes. The training analysts worked with their control analysands and received direction from more experienced analysts. Today, supervision can be received at various times throughout a clinician's career: during training, during the beginning of practice and during difficult times in the therapeutic process (e.g. impasses, etc.). All professionals who practice psychotherapy and/or counselling receive supervision during their training and are strongly encouraged to obtain clinical supervision after graduation. Supervision provides the opportunity for the therapist to review their work with an objective third party, who is often more experienced and educated about particular area(s) of psychotherapy. This third party can offer expression of the supervisor's response to the therapist, as well as that of the patient, and the possibility of unacknowledged feelings and behaviours. The supervisor is frequently chosen because the therapist admires the work of the supervisor and wishes to learn techniques and approaches, and, at the same time, resolve the difficulty in the casework. During my career as a music therapist, music therapy supervision following graduation was rare. Rarer still was the supervisor who was knowledgeable in psychotherapy and music therapy practices and procedures. Therefore, until recently, music therapists needed to obtain further education and supervision from verbal psychotherapists. Today, more music therapists with advanced training can provide the clinical assistance sought by practicing music therapists, as is done in other health care professions.

Clinical material

Ilene telephoned for an appointment for supervision by stating that she needed help on her first job. She stated that in addition to reviewing her ideas for a programme in a nursing home, she was worried about how to work with her boss. At the first meeting she focused on her anger and frustration over the 'demands' by her boss in relation to her hours, with which patients she could work, where she could work and storage of her equipment.

Over five sessions the therapist and I began reviewing her cases (one group and two individuals) and began to see a difference between the therapist's feelings about herself with her boss and herself with the patients. This awareness culminated in a piano improvisation that focused on finding what music would describe herself in these two situations. With this new awareness we could begin to concretize why her boss was stimulating the feelings of inability, worthlessness and inefficiency. The therapist and I were able to look at the therapist's specific attributes which might be contributing to this relationship. Manifestly, one aspect was a difference in response time and another was her insecurity about accurately producing the required paperwork describing her clinical work. As the therapist became more aware of how the boss' character style was similar to others who had caused difficulties in her life, we were able to develop strategies and responses to have available towards a variety of staff (particularly her boss).

We were also able to explore any similar reactions in the supervision setting in regard to self-deprecating comments prior to musically imitating a patient's responses or playing her own part in therapy sessions. This particularly affected her ability to problem solve at work and in the supervisory session. She often asked for solutions to problems, rather than use the supervision as a way to learn problem-solving. Again, this was a character trait that was creating difficulty for her as a part-time worker. As supervisor, I encouraged her to work in ways that were comfortable to her. However, urgent queries for help continued, though with less frequency. As we continued to look at the clinical processes, the therapist became more aware of how and why she was interacting verbally and musically with her patients. At times, her reluctance to express herself musically mirrored that of her patient. At those points, we looked at the thoughts behind the resistance for both the therapist and the patient. The imitation of the patient's musical, non-verbal and verbal responses during the supervision session provided opportunities to learn to make clinical judgements as the session proceeded. This reflective use of music was explored in terms of interpretations of possible communication of ideas or feelings in the moment about the therapist, the therapy or other therapy issues. The increased knowledge made it easier to complete the required paperwork, gain knowledge about her strengths (especially with this population) and her integration of knowledge about music therapy (as demonstrated by her increased attempts to use specific types of musical interventions for a variety of therapy issues).

Following a year of supervision, Ilene was able to successfully apply and receive her music therapy credentials. In addition, she gave an in-service on music therapy for the nursing home staff – after which she began to receive referrals from staff other than her boss. This reduced the dependence and amount of contact with her boss and opportunities for feedback from other staff. Ilene also exhibited increased ability to answer questions about her work spontaneously to nursing staff.

Theoretical framework

As a psychoanalytically oriented music therapist and supervisor, I organize my observations and acquisition of verbal and non-verbal information within the framework of psychodynamic theories, particularly object relations theory. Thus the basis of emotional distress involves internal conflict based on the consequences of the relationship between the primary caretaker (object) and the infant. As psychodynamic theory has been modified to include greater awareness and use of the therapist/patient relationship in reality and in a time-restricted fashion, so too have I tried to incorporate these ideas to my supervisees. However, the basic techniques of reflection and interpretation remain essential to my therapy and supervisory work. In addition, I use the developmental stage behaviours, based on the work of Erikson, Klein and Mahler, to understand the functioning of both the patient and the therapist. Psychodynamic theory is a stage theory. Therefore, a person is, theoretically, unable to proceed to a more mature developmental stage until the present one is successfully completed. The patient re-enacts his past relationships until the conflicts are resolved. D.W. Winnicott describes this work by the therapist as being a 'good enough mother' (Abram 1997). This term was first developed during the 1950s, but did not appear in Winnicott's writings until 1967–68 (Winnicott, Sheperd and Davis 1989). The supervisor inherits the role of object in the supervisory dyad. It can begin with the supervisor assuring the clinician that they are not 'losing their therapy skills' or 'bad therapists for having negative feelings towards their patients'. The supervisor then offers a place to confidentially look at what is occurring in the clinical setting and support the therapist in his attempt to begin to resolve the particular conflicted feelings that are contributing to emotional distress or affecting the therapist's clinical judgement. In this way the supervisor helps the therapist contain the anxieties stimulated by conflicts between internal and external environments. Therefore, taking the role of the 'good-enough mother' creates a holding environment for the anxieties and insecurities of the child (Winnicott 1972).

While numerous books and journals provide the description of object relations theory and practice (a good compilation of writings on object relations theory is in Buckley (1986)), I do not know of any literature in the music therapy field which is framed exclusively in this theory. However, under various other names which include the word 'analysis', similar descriptions of therapist and patient issues are described (e.g. Priestley and Tyson). Books on various aspects and ways to provide analytically oriented supervision have been written by Robert Langs (1994), Rock (1997), Clarkson (1998) and Lane (1990), and an entire volume of *Psychoanalytic Inquiry* is devoted to describing aspects of psychoanalytic supervision (Levy and Kindler 1995). Based on a psychoanalytic way of working, the therapist is encouraged to bring information to the supervision in her own way. How the information is presented offers the supervisor information about the therapist as well as the patient. For example: Does the therapist bring only information about certain aspects of the therapy process? Is she willing to look at her own role and feelings about the therapy situation? How does the presentation of the therapist imitate the presentation of the patient(s)? This information is obtained verbatim and also in behaviour between the supervisor and the therapist (e.g. Does the therapist always come to sessions prepared to perform and resistive to spontaneous exploration off the prepared track?). Thus exploring the transference and countertransference becomes a constant reflection of the triadic relationship between the patient, therapist and supervisor. Increasing the therapist's awareness of how the patient may use primitive defence mechanisms, which will affect the therapist's reactions and residual feelings following a therapy session, is frequently an important part of the supervisory work. Almost all authors on supervision admit that the role of supervisor is a multifaceted one. Mainly, there appear to be two major roles: one of teacher and one utilizing the supervisor's skills as a therapist.

Use of music in supervision

As free associations are important to psychoanalytically oriented verbal therapy, so music improvisation becomes an all-important means of acquiring information. While the supervisor needs to obtain certain verbal demographic information at the start, I also search for the first opportunity for musical facilitation and exploration. I try to demonstrate the musical concepts of reflection and interpretation (verbalizing the musical expression and musically expressing the verbal statements). I suggest that the clinician approach the task of supervision in any way they wish. At this point, he may also let me know what information he perceives as pertinent. From the beginning, I ask him to look at his affective reactions and responses. I also ask, during the 45-minute weekly session, to provide a processed session, where a therapy session is written in detail (e.g. he said..., she said..., I said). With this, we can begin to look at what is occurring in the therapy session as well as in the supervisory session. Most importantly, the thoughts prior to the therapist's responses can be addressed. The clinician also often tells me what they think is the problem and asks for alternative ideas. For example, a relatively experienced music therapist arranged for supervision. 'Suzanne' presented as a 'good supervisee' by coming to the sessions prepared to focus on why the previously used music therapy techniques were not working in a new work setting. As long as we stayed in verbal expression and addressed the specific techniques she used with therapy groups, there was no acknowledgement of repressed feelings towards her patients, who were substance abusers. The existence of countertransference issues were considered in her need to 'bend over backwards' to gratify various demanding group members. However, when she attempted to put her feelings in a piano improvisation, based on what it would feel like to lead the group, she was able to feel and recognize her anger in working with substance abuse patients and at the clinic staff (who replicated her dysfunctional family dynamic). We were then able to begin to look at the dynamics of the substance abuser and how the therapist can help them express these issues musically as well as verbally. In addition, she could help them recognize and understand their resistant behaviour of directing their anger onto the therapist and overwhelming her. After seven sessions she felt ready to work on her own again, with a new way of approaching the work with her patients and coping with the centre's organization. She also became more aware of unresolved issues about her work, which would be brought to her own therapy.

Frequently, music therapists seek supervision in order to increase their knowledge in relation to their work. They will describe their difficulty as being 'bored', 'hating to go to work' and 'feeling that their patients are losing interest or becoming hostile and/or inappropriate'. In other words, they convey the message that they have 'lost' their ability and/or enthusiasm to do clinical work. I often ask the therapist to imitate the patient's musical responses on instruments available in the supervision setting. Though musically accomplished, many music therapists find this a difficult task. Similar to resistance in the therapy setting (Austin and Dvorkin 1993), the ease in verbal description, as opposed to the musical one, becomes the first subject of exploration. I regard my role primarily as a teacher. However, many supervisees initially come to supervision in a distressed emotional state. Therefore, I find I need to learn a little about the therapist and their relationship to me and to their work before alternative ways of working can be discussed. This information will often relate to how they might use the information they receive in supervision. Because of the initial distress and intense anxiety, it is frequently difficult for the therapist to verbally describe his/her feelings about the therapy situation – that is, how do they feel about the patient, the therapy setting, the therapy material (latent and manifest) and their own work. Instead, the therapist may safely restrict themselves to a chronological description of what has already occurred at the workplace. This is where the use of music is most helpful in my practice.

The music therapist is asked to musically express (vocally and/or instrumentally) her feelings about the patient or setting. During this part, my role as supervisor becomes a combination of teacher and therapist – 'therapist' in that I will be listening to the supervisee as a therapist to learn about his/her relatedness to me and the patient, modelling how this type of interaction may be beneficial or inhibitory to the therapy work, and 'teacher' in helping the supervisee to learn how the choice of interaction is accomplished. Following the therapist's role that I take in my therapy work, I usually do not join the music. However, if the therapist is unable to play due to intense anxiety, I will supply a supportive, reflective accompaniment. If requested to do so, I ask the therapist what her preferences are in terms of this support (e.g. Is there a particular instrument you want me to use? Where do you want me to sit? etc.). When the therapist finishes improvising, there is a verbal discussion about the musical affective qualities and their relationship to the therapist's, now conscious, feelings. The music often provides a means of bringing unconscious associations to a conscious level. At this point, the therapist is often able to acknowledge previously unexpressed verbal responses about his work (individual patients as well as groups or entire clinical systems). As I verbalize any interpretations I may have about the musical expression (therapist role), I also point out where the impression came from in the music (teacher role). I attempt to convey how I integrated the musical expression, the therapist's behaviour and verbal expression, and knowledge about the clinical population/setting in order to offer ideas about what needs to be addressed during the supervision process. As complementary to the psychoanalytic technique, it is more productive for the therapist to discover these issues on his own. This is accomplished through guided questions from the supervisor and his own education about musical expression. This part of the process may take two to three weeks to begin, depending on the degree of resistance to personal musical expression.

As in the therapy process, exploration of the patient's and therapist's music is essential to understanding what is occurring. In addition, the relationship between the therapist and supervisor can also be a source of information, as in the concept of parallel process. The patient's behaviour with the therapist is re-enacted in the therapist's behaviour with the supervisor. Therefore, different aspects of this triadic relationship can be role played in a variety of ways. In music therapy supervision the focus I use when interpreting the music is similar to the therapist's in that I listen for discrepancies between behaviour, verbal and musical expression. I then point out these discrepancies in order to explore the transference/counter-transference issues. In this way I can begin to see how the relationship between the therapist and patient, and/or therapist and supervisor, is played out. The therapist who resists the use of music in the supervision session also expresses this discomfort to his patient. The effect of this anxiety can also be explored in the safety of the supervision session, as it applies to the therapy setting. At the same time, the therapist is being asked to listen to the patient in a different way. Frequently, an issue for the music therapist concerns performance ability in contrast to the patient's ability or expectations. This also becomes an issue for 'performing' in front of the supervisor (or her own therapist). As the supervisor/therapist, it is part of my job to help the therapist work on this countertransferential issue. However, I do stop at the point of recognition and suggest that the issue be brought up in the therapist's own therapy. The boundary between supervision and therapy can be very thin, due to the similarity in techniques and the enormous effect the therapist's own unresolved issues can have on the clinical work. As an analytically oriented music therapy supervisor, I do not further explore the primary or past relational experiences that have led to this behaviour. For me, this distinguishes therapy from supervision. However, it is often helpful to the therapist to suggest factors which could have affected his behaviour, as verbal therapists may not be educated about psychological relationships to music as reflective of developmental/emotional issues.

Why have supervision?

As the director of a music therapy training programme, as well as a clinician, I believe that supervision is vital to the growth of a clinician as well as the field of music therapy. The type of supervision changes based on the education level of the therapist. The supervision of a student includes not only increasing awareness of methods and techniques but also the need to increase the ability to see and hear their patients in different ways. As a new therapist, the tendency to only see the patient in one way, and thus respond to the patient in that way, is not unusual. Supervision, during an internship, often focuses on this type of exploration (e.g. What is another way to look at this person? What might be another way to handle this clinical situation? etc.). As the clinician becomes more experienced, he/she reaches a point where they have become comfortable utilizing the techniques they have learned and want to learn more about working with their patients, which might include learning different ways of working as well as more intensive knowledge about the patient population.

Often, there are only one or two music therapists in a clinical setting. This limits the opportunity for clinical music therapy discussion or feedback. The therapist's supervisor frequently assumes an administrative role, rather than clinical, due to training in a different profession. The acceptance of the need for supervision as a part of ongoing training contributes to the respect that is given to the professionals in other health fields. In practicing psychotherapy, supervision is really the only way (once basic theoretical knowledge is obtained) to learn the techniques. As previously stated, the verbal psychotherapy literature is tremendous. The literature describing music therapy/psychotherapy practice is growing from individual descriptions of methods to books which describe a variety of frameworks in which music therapists work (e.g. Bruscia 1991). No matter where music therapists are working, they are offering some sort of musical relationship within the therapy and, therefore, require a basic knowledge of psychotherapeutic techniques and frameworks. While the music therapist may be overtly utilizing methods and activity techniques, a lack of understanding about what is occurring between the therapist and the patient neglects at least two-thirds of what is happening. The result is either the patient or therapist dropping out of the relationship without understanding the difficulties that arose within and between these two individuals. I have not found any clinicians who have not encountered experiences such as these. As a supervisor, I consciously make an effort not to encourage imitation of my developed technique. Instead, I focus on teaching the therapist how to clinically assess and judge situations as they occur in the therapy process as well as investigate what type of interventions would be most helpful (given the particular patient and therapist). In the end the therapist often changes how they work overtly and covertly (their thinking process) and once again begins to feel excited about the career he/she has chosen. In addition, they have also learned about aspects of themselves and their effect on a therapist's work.

Glossary

'Good enough mother': 'A designation used to indicate a mother who offers a holding environment which provides an optimal amount of constancy and comfort for the infant who is wholly dependent on her...She offers it at the 'right time' instead of imposing her own timing and needs. Then, when the infant must face frustration, aggression and loss, she also provides support within a setting of ongoing basic empathy and holding' (Moore and Fine 1990, p.205).

'Parallel process': '...the transferential pattern emergent in the analysand – analyst relationship is re-created in the analyst-supervisor relationship through the presentation of the clinical material. In other words, the supervisor's experience of the analyst "reflects" the relationship that is occurring between analysand and analyst' (Rock 1997, p.192).

References

Abram, J. (1997) *The Language of Winnicott.* Northvale, NJ: Jason Aronson Inc.

Austin, D. and Dvorkin, J. (1993) 'Resistance in individual music therapy.' *The Arts In Psychotherapy 20*, 5, 423–429.

Bruscia, K. (ed) (1991) *Case Studies in Music Therapy.* Phoenixville: Barcelona Publishers.

Buckley, P. (ed) (1986) *Essential Papers on Object Relations.* New York: New York University Press.

Clarkson, P. (ed) (1998) *Supervision - Psychoanalytic and Jungian Perspectives.* London: Whurr Publishers.

Lane, R. (ed) (1990) *Psychoanalytic Approaches to Supervision.* New York: Brunner/Mazel.

Langs, R. (1994) *Doing Supervision and Being Supervised.* London: Karnac Books.

Levy, J. and Kindler, A. (eds) (1995) *Special Issue on 'Psychoanalytic Supervision'. Psychoanalytic Inquiry.* Vol. 15, 2. Hillsdale: The Analytic Press.

Moore, B. and Fine, B. (eds) (1990) *Psychoanalytic Terms and Concepts.* New Haven: Yale University Press.

Rock, M. (ed.) (1997) *Psychodynamic Supervision.* Northvale: Jason Aronson.

Winnicott, C., Sheperd, R. and Davis, M. (eds) (1989) *Psychoanalytic Explorations of D.W. Winnicott.* Cambridge: Harvard University Press.

Winnicott, D. (1972) *Holding and Interpretation.* New York: Grove Press.

Suggested reading

Glickauf-Hughes, C. and Wells, M. (1997) *Object Relations Psychotherapy.* Northvale: Jason Aronson Inc.

Greenberg, J. and Mitchell, S. (1983) *Object Relations in Psychoanalytic Theory.* Cambridge: Harvard University Press.

Scharff, J. and Scharff, D. (1995) *The Primer of Object Relations Therapy.* Northvale: Jason Aronson Inc.

CHAPTER 15

Music Therapy Training
A Process to Develop the Musical and Therapeutic Identity of the Music Therapist

Tony Wigram, Jos De Backer and Jan Van Camp

Introduction

Training music therapists to a satisfactory musical, clinical and academic level is a complex and difficult task. The results of the WEK survey of 1993 (a questionnaire survey on the content of music therapy courses designed by Wigram, Erdonmez and Kortegaard) revealed that training courses in music therapy in Europe generally agree on the importance of grounding courses in psychology and music therapy methods, but there were considerable differences between courses as to how much time was devoted to education in the areas of musical skills, medical studies, clinical practice and personal development, and to what depth. This survey was very comprehensive and 41 questionnaires were returned, which represented a 50 per cent response. Courses in some countries were sampled and different models have emerged. In the United Kingdom, Sweden and Norway post-graduate study lasting between one and two years full-time is uniform, following a three-year or more music degree or equivalent. In the Netherlands the model developed through a combined arts therapies education programme at high-school level, with a specialization in music therapy. Germany, France and Finland have a variety of courses, generally three years in length. In Belgium and Denmark the university-based courses are both five-year full-time programmes. Part-time courses are more typical in Spain and Italy, where training can vary between two and four years (Wigram, Erdonmez and Kortegaard 1993; Erdonmez 1995).

Cheryl Dileo identified three important themes in music therapy education:

1. What are the skills, knowledge, abilities and qualities necessary for the practice of music therapy?

2. How are these skills taught?

3. How effectively, and with what degree of accountability, are these skills taught?
(Maranto 1987)

These questions not only address what the student is supposed to be learning but also who is teaching and how the quality of their teaching is monitored. This leads naturally to questions about the content of music therapy courses and, in order to address the issue of accountability, the need for independent, external examination as a form of quality control.

There has been much discussion in Europe about the potential for establishing a common standard for music therapy education. This has proven very difficult, given the wide variation in the length of training courses – from a one-year post-graduate study to five-year full-time studies – and the variation in the content of courses. In order to establish such a standard, we could use the model of competency based evaluation, as developed in the USA and documented recently by Sandness (1994), together with a primary criteria for what is included, or should we try to achieve more agreement about the areas of study and clinical experience included in the curriculum?

We would like to look at this from the perspective of the identity of the music therapist. We want to focus on aspects of their training that provides them with a therapeutic identity and the parts that develop their musical identity and personal resources.

What makes a good music therapist? It is interesting that in a study by Shatin, Kotter and Longmore in the USA (1968), attributes for a 'successful' music therapist were found to be:

- more outgoing (significant)

- concrete in their thinking

- intelligent

- somewhat submissive and mild

- sensitive

- self-sufficient.

As a result of different models of training, and within the different models of training, there are a number of dichotomies and contradictions, especially when trying to make decisions about the best use of the limited time for training to establish priorities:

- eclectic understanding and model versus single philosophical standpoint and method
- musical skills in piano and voice versus additional training in other instruments, including other first-study instruments
- focus on improvisational approaches versus inclusion of music repertoire, receptive approaches and structured musical activities
- supervised clinical practice during the course versus post-course internships under supervision
- allowing and nurturing the students to develop their own individual approach versus requirement that they develop skills within an existing method.

Another important aspect to consider is the quality and resources of the teachers. Typically, there are one or two, or, at most, three, experienced music therapists involved at a full-time level on a training programme. They tend to be specialized in one, possibly two, areas. Therefore, music therapy programmes involve many part-time teachers in teaching elements of the curriculum in which the full-time teachers or head of studies have either no expertise or no time to do it themselves. Clinicians from other disciplines, and music specialists, are brought in to teach as part-time teachers.

Subjects often taught by non-music therapists on courses include: psychology, medicine, anatomy/physiology, theory of therapy, research skills, statistics, psychiatry, pathology, piano, guitar, improvisation, music analysis, voice, notation and basic music skills.

In clinical practice there is supervision by non-music therapists and, in personal development: individual therapy, group therapy, and group dynamics.

Subjects usually taught by music therapists include: music therapy theory, music therapy methods, clinical improvisation, music psychology and music therapy as a psychotherapeutic method.

The advantage of such a variety of input into a programme is the richness and intensity of many different 'experts'. The disadvantage is the confusion generated by so many different elements, especially if the central process of development is not co-ordinated or integrated. We all have a wish to provide students with as comprehensive a training as possible and try to make a balance between all the different elements to ensure that the student, at the end of a training course, feels:

- academically and scientifically grounded
- musically skilled in performance competency and improvisational flexibility
- medically knowledgeable
- clinically experienced and confident
- professionally competent to undertake, evaluate, analyse and report
- ethically informed
- personally stable and secure
- therapeutically insightful, empathic and intuitive.

This is our ambition.

The development of a therapeutic and musical identity is achieved by the connection and integration of these elements through three main processes:

1. Therapy: therapeutic understanding and insight

2. Art: musical skills in clinical application

3. Science: academic, clinical and professional competence.

The university programmes in music therapy at Aalborg University and Leuven University/Lemmensinstituut – both five-year, full-time Masters level programmes in music therapy – have struggled with the problem of balancing all these elements and we shall use these programmes as models for our discussion on the theme of developing the musical and therapeutic identity of the music therapists in a training course.

Therapeutic identity

From the previous outline of the curriculum of the music therapist's training, it becomes obvious that the candidate, in accordance with the two parts of the term 'music therapy', needs to be well grounded in the field of music as well as in the field of psychotherapy. The component 'therapy' functions as predicate ('this musician is a therapist') suggests that the professional identity of the music therapist is not primarily derived from his education at the conservatoire but, rather, comes about within his therapeutic formation and the socio-professional framework of the mental health care in which he is active.

The social definition and allocation of this profession holds the danger that the artistic component is rather considered as an incidental circumstance which has a purely utilitarian character within the scope of a mainly therapeutic activity. Making music is only of importance in so far as it serves a therapeutic objective. Even though his assignment is therapeutic and he commits himself to the ethics of vocational work, the question remains as to whether or not the music therapist harms the nature of art and the task of the artist through this professional identification and the reduction of the artistic process to a medium of therapeutic action.

A first starting point on this issue is the question: 'For what reasons do the students choose to train in music therapy?'

Motivation and choice for music therapy

We have noticed that there are two types of students who have chosen music therapy training. On the one hand there are students who have completed an education at the conservatoire, through which they have gradually discovered that their vision of and contact with music brought them closer to the kind of music practice as it takes shape in music therapy, rather than going the way for which they were predestined by their training – that is, to become a music teacher or a performing musician.

On the other hand there are students who do have a good musical training but only choose a professional music course because of the direct motivation to become a therapist. Many of them would have chosen another job in vocational work if their love for music was not as important.

Intuitively, we would say that the traditional reasons that have a part in choosing a profession within vocational work are more openly present in the latter group. The former group consists of musicians who have many affinities with a music practice that is characterized as 'musica practica' by Roland Barthes.

'Musica practica' is a style of making music as done by the perfect amateur – not so much aimed at the auditive and euphony (and in what follows: the concert, the record, the radio) but manual, muscular, physical and performed in a studio (not for an audience) where music is made with other people. Historically, this style is almost extinct, but music therapists consider themselves as the heirs of this music making – that leads more to acting than listening. Reducing the requirement to achieve polished sounds and expression does not mean giving up technical perfection. A great technical competence is, for obvious reasons, also a condition to free one's self of codes of expression that kill the listener's own activity. Probably, it is likely that students have undertaken a complete musical training to discover this affinity with practical music, but a sufficient familiarity with professional music practice seems essential to us before a final choice is made for music therapy. This training frustrates the student for two years in his therapeutic aspirations and compels him to use this time for mainly musical study. The focus on music and the constraint of therapeutic eagerness must emphasize a well-considered choice after the undergraduate years. The love of music is essential.

Is the music therapist an artist?

By stating that love of music needs to be a decisive factor in the choice of the candidate, we not only want to point to the sources he draws from to form his professional identity but we also want to make it clear that these sources are indispensable to irrigate the ground on which the therapeutic activity itself takes roots.

Each therapeutic activity is embedded in a framework which supports the dual relationship between patient (or group of patients) and therapist. This framework refers to the more or less institutionalized collection of attitudes, convictions, ideas and practices that are shared by a group of music therapists.

A therapist does not reinvent psychotherapy for himself in an arbitrary way. However intimate the relationship with his client may be, the therapist always appears as a representative of a group that stands for a particular way of thinking and acting. This shared framework preserves every therapeutic relationship from falling into a pure mimetism of an imaginary nature.

The technique and the special relationship that this process establishes enables the client to transfer to the therapist that from which he suffers – his unconscious attitudes and his fantasies. The client relies on the therapist, representing and guaranteeing a knowledge and a skill, to integrate all of his suffering in a meaningful context.

To establish a confidential transfer (surrender) at the level of making music, it is necessary that the person to whom one expresses himself spontaneously and unconditionally is so familiar with the material that he even succeeds in responding to the most bizarre and incomprehensible forms. Mind you, responding not in the sense of interpreting or attaching one or other psychological meanings to it but responding within a context (unity) of tradition that has explored these forms. It is a current clinical observation that the musical expressions (utterances) of patients are richer, more refined, more differentiated and of a higher aesthetic standard as the therapist makes use of higher professional skills. Just as a patient only brings up these elements that have received an accessible place in the psyche of the therapist, in music therapy only these musical forms get a chance to which the music therapist is *de facto* and, in principle, receptive.

From the obvious idea that every music therapy session can only claim to be a therapeutic activity if, in its starting point and objective, it is defined as an artistic activity, the focus on this aesthetic dimension in the formation of the student is essential. The distinction with verbal psychotherapy does not lie in the fact that in arts therapies the medium happens to shift from a verbal to a musical or pictorial language but that arts therapies are basically determined by their artistic, fictional, artificial and playful character. Music therapy derives its strength from appearance. Even to the clients who enjoy a traditional and obviously preferential treatment with music therapists – that is, those who are deprived of verbal language (in autism or dementia, etc.) – music therapy does not offer in the first place an alternative language but the possibility to obtain access, through fictionalizing, to their mental reality or to reality *überhaupt.*

The real mission of the music therapist lies in the ability to play with the material that he owns. He needs to have a passion for music, to stay in touch with music in all its forms and especially with contemporary music. In the same way as our time takes shape in the authentic music that is now written, social and cultural trends enter the forms in which psychopathology manifests itself now.

The development of the psychotherapeutic identity is as equally important a cornerstone as the development of the musical identity. The way in which music is handled in a therapeutic setting is embedded in a specific therapeutic background. We do develop analytically orientated music therapists. Our starting point is psychoanalysis translated into a particular psychotherapeutic method, and which is, at the same time, an anthropology because it has a specific vision on man. Research is not possible without a life-science theory. We always need an anthropological frame of reference. From the psychoanalytic way of thinking, a method or approach is developed from the basis by which the therapist deals with the musical material of the patient. It is essential that a space is created where the patient, through his musical expressions, discovers things about himself of which he was not previously aware.

Psychoanalysis is not primarily aimed at direct recovery (healing). The analyst's main concern is not to cure the patient of depression or anxiety. The music therapist cannot remove a depression by applying certain musical means or ease a handicap with specific music. What matters is that the patient can express himself in musical improvisations, that musical speaking is enabled, that the patient gets a space in which he can make music and that through this music making certain elements can appear that surprise him, of which he was not previously aware. This is the essence of analytical therapy – create a space within which experiences can originate, experiences that can be linked to images and words. Without images and words to replace the musical experience, this experience keeps its characteristic properties in its aesthetic form.

So the music therapist works in a psychotherapeutic way, not necessarily in a verbal way but at a pre-verbal, non-verbal or supra-verbal level, through music. Nevertheless, (s)he needs to have an understanding of psychological processes. As a therapist, (s)he is charged with the care of the patient. (S)he works within a context, a team for which the therapeutic aspect is essential. (S)he needs to give a place to the sometimes bizarre expressions (utterances) of the patient.

A theoretical background is important. The student needs to be sufficiently able at an intellectual level to develop satisfactory knowledge in subjects such as psychopathology, psychiatry, developmental psychology, music and society, depth psychology, etc.

Music therapy self-experience

A therapeutic training cannot only consist of an enumeration of skills and techniques. A student has to experience the process him/herself. Music therapy or psychotherapeutic self-experience is obvious. We expect from the applicant music therapy student the willingness to work on him/herself and a personal engagement in the training, during which (s)he follows his/her own therapy. This also holds for the lecturers and professors. For that matter, students can feel perfectly well whether their lecturers have their own therapeutic experience behind them or whether they have gone through a therapeutic process. If they have not done so, they cannot pass on the therapeutic process in an adequate way. So it is obvious that music therapists go through their own therapeutic experience. There are many reasons for this and we would like to go more deeply into one of them. Transference is one of the most important phenomena in a therapeutic relationship and students need to experience it.

Transference, which is present in every human relationship, and also, for example, in the musical ensemble of an orchestra or chamber orchestra, achieves a special significance in a music therapy setting. Transference is only possible when the music therapist takes up a reserved position, so that the patient can use him for transfer of central persons and relationships in his life. Differing from other relationships, these transference phenomena are raised by the abstinence of the therapist. It is even essential for the therapy that these images of father or mother can be made conscious. The projection of these images of central figures on the therapist, and the recurrence of these relationships within the therapeutic relationship, is defined by Freud as 'transference neurosis'. The development and continuing effect of this transference neurosis is an essential component of the therapeutic process. Only when the music therapist takes up a reserved and neutral position, even in his musical play, does he create the possibility to incarnate the conflicts and ambivalences of the patient and to continue working on them through discussion.

What does discussion mean in music therapy? How does the music therapist deal with psychological elements and conflicts of which the patient was not aware before and which come up in music therapy sessions?

This discussion primarily comes about through the so-called musical reflection. The therapist tries to linger over and think through the spontaneous emotional reactions that arise in himself and with the patient in the sessions. These reactions are particularly significant if they are given a musical form by the therapist in an alluding or confronting way and are experienced by the patient as bizarre or surprising.

The musical retention and repetition of such themes at the right moment contribute to the fact that the patient can arrogate these unconscious but staged contents when he is ready to. That is why it is so important that students go through their own therapeutic process and can experience these transfer phenomena in order to acquire an understanding of their abilities and limits, both psychologically and musically. We believe that the training has to provide a basis from which the student can build his own specific therapeutic identity, in which he gets the space to experience how he will handle musical materials in his music therapy practice. The training needs to provide a clear point of reference from which the students can start.

Identity of the training

There are music therapy trainings that start from several psychotherapeutic methods which are being discussed and acquired. These are the so-called eclectic trainings. But once you graduate, what do you represent? Models can become fragmented.

A patient may need to know which therapy model his therapist works with and in which frame of reference he places his materials. This is the basis for the trustworthiness of a therapeutic relationship. What is a therapist without a personal vision? We do agree if people reproach us for seeing everything through 'tinted glasses', but we prefer tinted glasses over incomplete, 'misty glasses', through which we can't see clearly. Yet, there is nothing to stop us from looking at other directions. From the analytical frame of reference, other models can be discovered. Within projects there is space to get to know these models through experience and to discuss them. During the foundation of a training it is valuable to organize project weeks and invite specialists to inform about different models. Then students have information at first hand of people who think within other models. This confrontation with other models is important from the interdisciplinary point of view. Students need to be well informed about different models and able to relate to them.

Balance

The two cornerstones of the training are the development of the musical and of the therapeutic identity, and they need to be in balance. In the course of the training the focus will be put on one then on the other cornerstone, so that students reach a balance of these two aspects.

Music skills in the music therapy training

There is no doubt that the recognition of music therapy as a profession relies upon its reputation as a 'specialized' intervention requiring the skills of a trained and unique professional.

In music therapy training courses different emphasis is placed on musical ability, both on entry and at final examinations and qualification. In some courses there is a focus on repertoire skills, the ability to play songs, using the guitar or piano, and the use of music in a functional or pedagogic way. Musical skills are evaluated through a mechanism of testing musical knowledge and competencies of performance.

Other traditions work through creative improvisation, and the therapist's musical skills are continuously assessed, and they are particularly evaluated in the context of clinical application.

Musical identity

But we can't just be satisfied with some accepted standard or level of performance. We can try to set criteria for good piano, improvisation or vocal skills and define what pieces, songs, accompaniments students should be able to play. But the *real* skill in music therapy that is most needed is the ability to be a 'musical being' in the session. We have to create a musical environment – presence – atmosphere. Our musical responses must be fine-tuned, natural, immediate, sensitive, appropriate. Our musical awareness must be wide ranging, founded on a broad base of experience, and at least some knowledge of the many different genres and styles of the last thousand years.

If we expect to train students to find a way of 'reaching, helping and healing' people who have a wide variety of disorders, handicaps or illnesses, these students must have a chameleon musical persona, fashioned round a strong, individual but flexible musical identity.

So what does this mean in practice in terms of how we can train students? What can you learn, and what is inborn and cannot be learned?

The two most important facilities are to hear and understand and to play with meaning. This is rather simplistic, but it is the essence. On top of both of these essential elements is a whole structure of abilities, skills, knowledge, experience and therapeutic sensitivity. It is a process which includes the process of developing your own musical identity, which connects with your therapeutic identity, the combination of which provides you with your professional identity.

The musical training in a music therapy programme, from the point of view of these two elements, needs to take into consideration the following necessary studies.

Music psychology

Form and analysis of musical structure:

- sonata, binary, ternary, rondo, theme and variations, minuet, etc.

- psychoacoustics
- anatomy of hearing
- acoustics
- repertoire
- vocal training
- use of voice with accompaniment
- body and voice
- facility with instruments
- guitar
- percussion
- musical dictation
- auditory training
- transposition
- harmonization
- composition
- extemporization
- modulation
- prima vista
- playing from chordal scoring, full scoring
- listening skills
- musical history
- major composers, performers
- a range of different music – classical, popular and folk
- an understanding of musical structure for emotional purposes
- programme music
- compiling a tape with a selection for a specific purpose
- songwriting.

What is the musical identity of the music therapist?

What is the musical identity of the music therapist?

Historically developed

- inborn musical aptitude
- history of musical experiences
- likes and dislikes in music – emotional reactions to music
- knowledge of different musical genres
- musical education
- identity through their skills and performance on their main instrument.

Developed in music therapy education

- improvisational flexibility
- awareness of meaning within music
- techniques for responding to clients' music, e.g. mirroring, matching, exaggerating, reflecting
- integration of their own musical history, experiences, likes.

Are we trying to develop the student's role and therapeutic personality as an artist? Is that the feeling therapists have when they are in sessions – I am perceived by clients and by my colleagues as an artist or a musician? Do we train students to allow their own musical identity to be evident in the therapeutic relationship? We hope so!

There is often a discussion – perhaps, an argument – about the need for the music therapist to have well-developed, sophisticated and expert musical skills. Students quickly become seduced by their psychotherapeutic role, by the power they gain from knowledge about things that are medical, scientific, clinical – knowledge about the history and problems of the clients with whom they are working. These elements in the training are essential for balance but can reduce the influence and importance of musical skill and the place of the therapist's musical identity in therapy.

So, when students at different levels of musical skill work at instrumental and vocal skills in transposition, harmonization, extemporization, rhythmic and melodic variability, as well as enlarging and expanding their knowledge of composed music, they may question the need for this in a way that could be an unconscious denial or resistance to accepting their own musical limitations and the need to develop. Why do I need to be able to do that? Doesn't working with free improvisation in music therapy mean I can break free from all the rules, structure, form and technical skills of conventional performance and musical training?

Well, whether we are using free improvisation or composed music in music therapy, the subtlety of how we work with musical material relies on a high level of skill and all-round knowledge.

We need to be very skilful and eclectic musicians. The music our clients bring into our sessions can range from:

- chaotic to structured
- simple to complex
- free improvisation to pre-composed songs
- baroque to modern jazz
- classical to romantic.

Our ability to understand our clients through their music depends on our own musical sensitivity, skill and experience. Attaching meaning to clients' musical material is achieved by:

- being able to listen to their music
- being able to remember and/or notate their music
- being able to analyse their music
- being able to contextualize their music
- being able to interpret the meaning within their music.

Up to the point of interpretation, the previous four stages require musical knowledge, education, skill and experience. The process described above applies equally to the therapist's music and, in mutual improvisation, to both the client's and the therapist's parts taken together. The contextualization and interpretation is where the integration of music and therapy takes place and can be unfounded and inadequate without the informed musical analysis.

In Aalborg, Denmark and the Lemmensinstituut, Belgium, time is given to asking students to describe musical material in musical terminology, to be able to vocally or instrumentally recall clients' musical themes and style of playing and to describe their own playing as a musical response. A particular focus is given to the way musical material from the client or the therapist changes over time, within an improvisation or within a whole session.

Transitions occur, representing change both in the music and in the pathological state of the client. Developing those transitions musically can be one of the most important skills of the music therapists – and it is a musical skill.

There is also discussion about how directive or non-directive the music therapist can be. Words with negative connotations such as 'manipulative', 'dominating' and 'structuring' are sometimes used to describe the approach of a therapist who is more directive. This also relates to the simplicity or complexity of the music. Using more sophisticated musical skills to frame your client's more simple music and establish your musical identity can be viewed as directive, but it can also be seen as containing, holding, inspiring and creative. The skills students need to acquire is to have such a high level of musical fluency that they can easily find a balance between following and initiating, symbiosis and independence, musical freedom and musical structure.

It is the balance of these elements, the combining of a number of different parts together to make the whole and reach the client, that can be premeditated, intuitive, adaptive, contrived, reactive or just sensitive and flexible. In the training of music therapy students there is a need to provide some clear framework for working in music therapy and to help them sort out the elements they can use and how they should be appropriately combined to the best effect in working with different problems.

There is no doubt that compared with other professionals, where there already exists a fairly clear understanding of their role and therapeutic value, music therapists are still faced everyday with fundamental questions:

- Why should I refer a client for music therapy?
- What are the aims and objectives of your therapy?
- What do you do in music therapy sessions?
- How do you evaluate if music therapy is helping the client?

A recently qualified music therapist needs to be able to answer these questions just as well as an experienced clinician, and offer a framework based on an integration of musical and therapeutic process.

In the end, when you are working with a psychotherapeutic approach in music therapy, you can only plan or prepare to a limited degree. In the session, when events happen and issues come up, we find ourselves drawing on our intuition and experience to find the way. Because of this need for creative flexibility, high-level musical skill, adaptable and creative improvisation skill, a sensitive musical and therapeutic identity are essential. This is what we should work with in music therapy education when training students.

References

Erdonmez, D. (1995) *Music Therapy Training Courses Directory: World Federation of Music Therapy*. Melbourne: Melbourne University.

Maranto, C. (1987) 'Continuing themes in the literature on music therapy education and training.' In C.Maranto and K. Bruscia (eds) *Perspectives on Music Therapy Education and Training*. Philadelphia: Temple University.

Sandness, M. (1994) 'National Association for Music Therapy: Standards and procedures for academic program approval.' *Music Therapy Perspectives 12*, 1, 39–50.

Shatin, L., Kotter, W. and Longmore, G. (1968) 'Personality profile of successful music therapists.' *Journal of Music Therapy 5*, 111–113.

Wigram, T., Erdonmez, D. and Kortegaard, H. (1993) *The WEK Questionnaire of Music Therapy Education*. Unpublished Questionnaire.

The Contributors

Sandra Brown, A.R.C.M., B.Mus (Edin), B.A. (Psych.), Dip.M.T. (N-R), trained as a music therapist at the Nordoff–Robbins Music Therapy Centre, London, and has worked with a wide range of clients. At present, she works as Senior Music Therapist at the centre and as Senior Clinical Tutor on the Master of Music Therapy degree course run by the centre. She also maintains a private supervision practice. She is currently training as a Jungian analyst with the Society of Analytical Psychology in London.

Jos De Backer, Dip. M.Th., studied music in Leuven, Belgium and music therapy in Vienna. He is Professor at the College of Science and Art at the Lemmensinstituut (Leuven) of Music Therapy and Coordinator for the training course in Music Therapy. He is Head of the Music Therapy Department at the University Centre, Kortenberg, where he works as a music therapist, treating young psychotic patients. He also has a private practice. He was organizing Chairman, and co-chairman of the Scientific Committee of the 4th European Music Therapy Conference in Belgium, 1998. He is Chairman of the 'Foundation Music and Therapy', and Vice-President of the European Music Therapy Confederation (EMTC). He is currently undertaking PhD research on the international PhD programme in Music Therapy at the University of Aalborg, Denmark. He specializes in psychoanalytically oriented music therapy, and has presented various papers and workshops on music therapy with handicapped people and psychiatric patients.

Janice M. Dvorkin, Psy.D., ACMT, is presently the co-ordinator of the Music Therapy Program at the University of the Incarnate Word, in San Antonio, Texas. She was Past President of the American Association for Music Therapy and is presently a member of the Assembly of Delegates in the American Music Therapy Association. She has practiced as a music therapist for 19 years and as a licensed psychologist for 6 years. Her work, with an emphasis on borderline personality disorder and object relations theory (as it effects clinical and supervisory work) has been presented nationally and internationally as well as published in books and journals. She maintains a clinical supervision practice for music therapists and is on the editorial board of the *Journal of Music Therapy*.

Pauline Etkin, Dip.P.P.Ed., Dip.M.T. (N-R), is Director of the Nordoff–Robbins Music Therapy Centre in London and Head of the two-year Master's Degree course at the centre. She also works clinically with children with a wide range of difficulties as well as with adults with learning difficulties. She is a member of the advisory council of the Association of Professional Music Therapists, serves as a committee member of the Courses Liaison Committee and the Supervision Core Panel of the APMT, and is a music therapy representative on the newly formed Arts Therapy Board which deals with state registration.

Claire Flower B.Mus (Man.), Dip.M.T., (GSMD), trained at the Guildhall School of Music and Drama in London. Having worked in both adolescent and adult mental health, she now works primarily in an education setting with children with a wide range of special needs. She has established introductory music therapy courses for undergraduate music students at a number of music colleges, and is now a member of the music therapy teaching staff at both the Guildhall School of Music and the Nordoff–Robbins Music Therapy Centre. She also maintains a private clinical supervision practice.

Isabelle Frohne-Hagemann, Dr. Phil., is head of the post-graduate training course 'Integrative Music Therapy' at the European Academy for Psychosocial Health (Fritz Perls Institut). She also trains music therapists at different universities, and is a freelance music therapist, gestalt therapist and supervisor for music therapists in Berlin. Born 1947 in Hamburg, she studied educational sciences and French, music, music therapy, medicine and psychotherapy. She is a qualified teacher, qualified 'Heilpraktikerin' and qualified Integrative (Music and Gestalt) therapist and qualified supervisor. She worked for 15 years as an assistant professor at the Academy of Music in Hamburg (sensory awareness and corporal education; anatomy and physiology; group improvisation, rhythmical education).

Gianluigi di Franco is musician (vocalist) and Freudian-oriented psychiatrist. He is the founder and director of the Training Course for Music Therapists, ISFOM, Naples, since 1989 and AIAS, Cosenza, since 1996. He has been reconfirmed as president of CONFIAM (Italian Confederation of Music Therapy Associations) for the period 1997–2000. At international level he is the founder and president of the E.M.T.C. (European Music Therapy

Confederation) for the period 1998–2001 and World Federation of Music Therapy Council Member for Publications (1996–1999), where, in particular he takes care of the newsletter. He is also co-ordinator of the Music Therapy Department for Deaf Children at the Institute of Audiology (Faculty of Medicine, University of Naples) and adjunct professor of Music Therapy at the University Course for Speech Therapists, University of Naples.

Simon Keith Gilbertson, Dip.M.T., Dipl.M.Th., is head of the department of Music Therapy at Klinik Holthausen, Germany. He gained a Bachelor of Music at King's College, University of London, (B.Mus.Hons.), a Diploma in Music Therapy at Nordoff–Robbins Music Therapy Centre, London and Diploma in Music Therapy at Institut für Musiktherapie, Universität Witten/Herdecke. Following his studies at King's College, where he majored in Composition and Ethnomusicology, he went on to study music therapy at the Nordoff-Robbins Music Therapy Centre, London. He began his first year working with a wide spectrum of clients ranging from pre-school children to adults living with autism, physical handicap and mental handicap. After moving to Germany in 1994 to work in the Klinik Holthausen, a clinic for early rehabilitation following neurosurgery where he gained experience working with both children and adults, he completed the diploma course at the Universität Witten/Herdecke. He has been Head of the Music Therapy Department for the past four-and-a-half years and has given papers on various aspects of neurosurgical rehabilitation in Rome, Boston and London.

Wendy Magee, PhD, is Head of Music Therapy, Royal Hospital for Neuro-disability, London. She was trained as a music therapist at the University of Melbourne, Australia, before moving to England nine years ago. Since 1990 she has worked at the Royal Hospital with adults who have complex neuro-disabilities stemming from severe or profound head injuries, stroke, Multiple Sclerosis or Huntington's disease. She has just completed doctoral research at the Department of Music, University of Sheffield. This has compared song and improvisation in clinical music therapy with individuals living with chronic neurological illness. In 1999 she will be acting Director to the MA in Music Therapy at the University of Limerick, Ireland.

Monika Nöcker-Ribaupierre, Dr.sc.mus., Dipl.Conductor (Munich), Dipl.MT (Hochschule für Musik und Theater, Hamburg), DBVMT, has undertaken research (University Children's Hospital Munich) into auditive stimulation after prematurity (Dr.sc.mus. 1994, Hamburg), music therapy with developmentally disabled children (University Children's Hospital and private practice) and auditive stimulation in NICU, Munich-Harlaching Hospital. She is head of Music Therapy Training in Munich, chair of the professional organization DBVMT and German co-ordinator of the EMTC (European Music Therapy Confederation). She has published a book and several articles.

Helen Shoemark is a music therapist at the Royal Children's Hospital, Melbourne, Australia. She completed her music therapy training at the University of Melbourne and Kansas University. Prior to moving into the clinical field of paediatrics and neonatology, Helen was known for her clinical work with children who have profound multiple disabilities. Helen taught in the music therapy programme and co-ordinated clinical training at the University of Melbourne for four years. She is immediate past President of the Australian Music Therapy Association (AMTAInc.) and registration advisor to the National Registration and Education Board of that organization.

John Strange, BA, DipEd, DipMTh, RMTh, ARCO, ARCM has been employed since 1986 as a music therapist in special schools. He has chaired the Association of Professional Music Therapists and currently represents the UK on the European Music Therapy Confederation and chairs the Committee for Arts Therapists in Education. He is becoming known as an expert witness on music therapy in paediatric medical injury legal cases.

Ann Turry, MA, CMT, NRMT, holds a Master's Degree from New York University and advanced clinical certification in Nordoff-Robbins Music Therapy. She served as a member of the Board of Directors of the American Association for Music Therapy for eight years, is currently on the board of directors of the Mid-Atlantic Region of the American Music Therapy Association and is a member of the Assembly of Delegates. She has presented internationally on music therapy with hospitalized children and has published a paper about music therapy in the medical procedure room. She supervises music therapy interns at Tomorrows Children's Institute and maintains a private teaching practice in New York City. Ann currently works at Tomorrows Children's Institute at Hackensack University Medical Center with chronically and terminally ill children.

Jan Van Camp is Professor at the College of Science and Art at the Lemmensinstituut and Coordinator of the training course for Music Therapy in Leuven. He is psychotherapist at the Univerity Centre, St Jozef, Kortenberg and supervisor/psychoanalyst at the Catholic University in Leuven. He was General Chairman of the 4th European Music Therapy Conference in Belgium, 1998.

Melanie Voigt, Ph.D., is head of the music therapy department at the Kinderzentrum München in Munich, Germany. She received a Bachelor of Music in Music Education from Texas Lutheran College, a Master of Music from Ithaca College and a Ph.D. in Music Education from the University of Texas at Austin. In 1984 she trained in Orff Music Therapy under Gertrud Orff at the Kinderzentrum München. Since that time she has worked using Orff Music Therapy in the treatment of children and youth with developmental disabilities. She is involved in co-ordinating training courses in Orff Music Therapy held at the Deutsche Akademie für Entwicklungs-Rehabilitation in Munich and is involved in the Ständige Ausbildungsleiterkonferenz Musiktherapie in Germany.

Tony Wigram, Ph.D., is Professor of Music Therapy and academic co-ordinator of Ph.D. Studies in Music Therapy at Aalborg University, Denmark. He is Head III Music Therapist at the Harper House Children's Service, and Research Advisor to Health and Community Services, both at Horizon NHS Trust, Hertfordshire, England. He is President of the World Federation of Music Therapy, and has positions as adjunct professor in music therapy on programmes in Italy, Spain and Belgium. He was a founder and co-ordinator/President of the European Music Therapy Confederation from 1989–1998. He travels and lectures extensively, has edited three books on music therapy, and published many articles.

Subject Index